The BMA guide to

RABIES

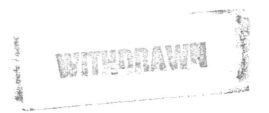

The BMA guide to

RABIES

Published on behalf of the British Medical Association by

Radcliffe Medical Press
Oxford and New York

Radcliffe Medical Press Ltd
18 Marcham Road, Abingdon, Oxon OX14 1AA, UK

Radcliffe Medical Press, Inc.
141 Fifth Avenue, New York, NY 10010, USA

British Library Cataloguing in Publication Data

A catalogue record for this book is available from the British Library.

ISBN 1 85775 180 9

Library of Congress Cataloging-in-Publication Data is available.

Typeset by MULTIPLEX medway ltd
Printed and bound in Great Britain

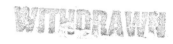

Contents

Editorial Board   viii

Board of Science and Education   ix

Working Party   x

Preface   xi

Acknowledgements   xiii

Glossary   xv

Chapter 1 Introduction: the threat of rabies   1
How rabies was eradicated from Britain   1
Quarantine in Britain   2
Rabies in Europe   4
Rabies outside Europe   5
Pasteur's experiments   5
The natural history of rabies   8
Rabies in animals   8
Rabies in man   12
Public attitudes to rabies, quarantine and change   17

Chapter 2 Current rabies legislation   19
Import of commercially traded animals from the EU   21
Responsibilities for preventing rabies in the UK   22

Chapter 3 Patterns of rabies around the world   25
Worldwide prevalence of rabies   25
Control of rabies around the world   26
Rabies-free countries using quarantine   27
Countries reporting no rabies   28

Chapter 4 Recent developments   39
The European Union   39
Development of oral vaccines for foxes and other animals   41
The Channel Tunnel   46

Chapter 5 Smuggling   51
Responsibility for control   51
Motives for smuggling   52

Chapter 6 Dealing with an outbreak of rabies in Britain   55
Understanding the threat of rabies   55
Potential sources for re-introducing rabies to Britain   57
Measures to control the fox population in a rabies outbreak   59
Predicting the pattern of rabies spread in Britain   63
Living with enzootic rabies in Britain   72

Chapter 7 Policy options for preventing rabies in Britain   74
How effective is quarantine?   75
Vaccination as a policy for rabies prevention   77

Chapter 8 Financial implications of various rabies policies   87
Costs of enzootic rabies in Britain   87
The cost of quarantine   90
Costs of a system of vaccination, certification and identification   90
Costs of eradication   91

Chapter 9 Reviewing the issues   92
The risk of rabies entering Britain   92
Rabies in Europe   93
Rabies and the threat to human life   94
The Channel Tunnel   95
The European Union   95
The consequences of rabies becoming endemic in Britain   96
The current system – advantages and disadvantages of
   quarantine   97
The alternative – vaccination and identification with
   serological testing   97
Smuggling   100
Financial considerations of different policies   101

Chapter 10 Recommendations: strategies for prevention and control   102
Two models for safeguarding Britain's future rabies-free status   102
The BMA's recommendations   105
Additional recommendations   107

Appendix I Rabies vaccines ancient and modern for human use   109
Vaccines prepared from nervous tissue   109
Vaccines prepared in avian embryos   110
Vaccines produced in cell cultures   110

Appendix II Vaccines for animals (including oral vaccination of foxes)   113
Vaccines prepared in avian embryos   113
Oral vaccines for foxes   113
Attenuated live rabies vaccines   113
Genetic recombinant vaccine   114

Appendix III Testing rabies vaccines   115
Mouse neutralization test (MNT)   116
Rapid fluorescent focus inhibition test (RFFIT)   116
Enzyme linked immuno sorbent assay (ELISA)   117

References   118

Index   131

Editorial Board

Board of Science and Education

This report was prepared under the auspices of the Board of Science and Education of the British Medical Association, whose membership for 1994/5 was as follows:

Working Party

The Board of Science and Education was advised by a working party whose membership was as follows:

Emeritus Professor of Medicine, University of Southampton; Chairman, BMA Board of Science and Education	*Professor J B L Howell (Chair)*
Director, Enteric and Respiratory Virus Laboratory, Central Public Health Laboratory	*Dr D W G Brown*
President, British Veterinary Association	*Mr C P DeVile*
Consultant in Communicable Disease Control, East Riding Health Authority	*Dr J M Dunlop*
Honorary Consultant, Public Health Medicine	*Dr P Grime*
Environmental Health Officer, Wood Green Animal Shelters, General Council member, Chartered Institute of Environmental Health	*Mr R L Leather*
Emeritus Professor of Anaesthesia, University of London	*Professor J Payne*
Director, The Centre for Tropical Medicine, Nuffield Department of Clinical Medicine, John Radcliffe Hospital, Oxford	*Professor D A Warrell*
Clinical Virologist	*Dr M J Warrell*

Preface

The British Medical Association's concern about rabies dates back to at least 1877. In that year a grant was made to investigate the natural history of rabies. Since then there have been many changes in the incidence, control and treatment of rabies worldwide, but it remains a disease which causes considerable fear and a high number of deaths in many areas of the world. In 1975, almost a century after the original research grant, the BMA expressed its concern about the dangers of smuggling animals, when its Annual Representative Meeting (ARM) passed the following motion:

> The Representative body is acutely aware of the danger of rabies being imported into the United Kingdom as the result of the irregular entry of dogs and certain other animals from the continent of Europe and calls for greater efforts to inform the public of the hazards involved in the evasion of quarantine restrictions.

Over the last twenty years scientific and political developments have prompted continuing discussion of the dangers of rabies. The desire to further the debate led to the Annual Representative Meeting of the BMA in 1992 passing a resolution:

> that the Board of Science and Education be requested to review the advantages and disadvantages of currently available methods of control and treatment of rabies; and to publicise its findings in order to inform the continuing debate on whether the present quarantine regulations should be maintained.

Acting on this, the Board of Science and Education, a standing committee of the Association, set up a Working Party to investigate this matter.

There are several events which have shaped the rabies discussion over recent years. The building of the first permanent physical link between

Britain and the European mainland, the Channel Tunnel, has led some to fear that rabies could travel to Britain via this route. The development of an effective oral vaccine to protect foxes against rabies has achieved considerable success in reducing the reservoir of rabies and has brought closer the prospect of a rabies-free Europe. This progress has been achieved through a European Union programme of vaccinating foxes, the main vectors of rabies in Europe.

As the European Union aims to harmonize its border controls, Britain's retention of its distinctive quarantine regulations has been questioned. If the oral vaccination programme succeeds in eliminating rabies from European Union countries, Britain's case for retaining its own different regulations will be weakened. Would it be necessary to retain such strict controls if the risk of rabies from these countries was reduced? Are there equally efficient methods of keeping Britain free from rabies which do not demand the expense and hardship of keeping a pet in quarantine for six months?

Changes to quarantine regulations are not just a matter for the future. Already the Ministry of Agriculture, Fisheries and Food (MAFF) has changed its regulations, in the light of Council Directive 92/65/EEC of 13 July 1992, known as the Balai Directive, on the import of animals for commercial trading. These animals may now enter Britain without quarantine if vaccinated, serologically tested, identified and accompanied by health certification. Many consider that public discussion of the issues is urgently needed.

Acknowledgements

The Association is indebted to the Working Party members for so generously giving of their time and expertise and is particularly grateful to the following organizations for their generous help and support in illustrating this publication:

British Small Animal Veterinary Association (BSAVA)
Eurotunnel
Hearing Dogs for the Deaf
Ministry of Agriculture, Fisheries and Food, Animal Health (Disease Control) A
Ministry of Agriculture, Fisheries and Food, © Crown copyright
Q A Photos © Eurotunnel
Rhône Mérieux
Professor D A Warrell
Dr M J Warrell
The Wellcome Centre/National Medical Slide Bank
The Wellcome Institute Library, London
The Wellcome Trust
World Health Organization
World Heath Organization Collaborating Centre for Rabies Surveillance and Research/Office International des Epizooties Reference Laboratory for Rabies, Tübingen

The Association is grateful for the specialist help provided by BMA Committees and many outside experts and organizations, and would particularly like to thank:

All the personnel in Animal Health (Disease Control) A, Ministry of Agriculture, Fisheries and Food; the late Mr Anthony Crowley, Veterinary Consultant to Eurotunnel; Dr Jack Done, Honorary Research Fellow, Agricultural Economics Unit, University of Exeter; Professor Stephen Harris, Professor of Environmental Sciences, School of Biological Sciences, University of Bristol; all the personnel in International Traffic Veterinary Control, Swedish Board of Agriculture; Dr Arthur King, formerly Rabies Research Leader, Central Veterinary

Laboratory, Weybridge; Professor J P McInerney, Agricultural
Economics Unit, University of Exeter; Dr Erik Millstone; the Rabies
Working Group of the Public Health Laboratory Service; Mr Kevin
Taylor, Assistant Chief Veterinary Officer, Ministry of Agriculture,
Fisheries and Food; Dr George S Turner, formerly Virologist, Lister
Institute of Preventive Medicine, Elstree; Dr Piran White, Lecturer in
Environmental Management, Department of Environmental Economics
and Environmental Management, University of York

Glossary

The terms below are defined in the context of the report

antibody
: complex protein (or immunoglobulin) found in the blood in response to the presence of an antigen. An antibody can attach to a particular antigen on an infectious organism and render it harmless (neutralization)

antigen
: substance which stimulates an immune response when introduced in an appropriate manner into a responsive animal. Rabies antigens are small parts of rabies virus proteins which can induce an immune response

attenuated virus
: a virus of reduced virulence

biomarker
: a label to show if an animal has been treated

booster vaccination
: a dose of vaccine given after a primary course to reawaken the immune response

carnivore
: a mammal adapted to eating flesh

compartmentation
: the restriction of an epizootic to a particular species

Creutzfeldt-jakob disease
: a fatal progressive disease affecting the central nervous system characterized by mental deterioration and loss of co-ordination of the limbs

cryptococcoetz
: a disease caused by the fungus *Cryptococcus neoformans* often affecting the central nervous system with meningitis

cytoplasm
: the contents of a cell contained within the cell membrane excluding the nucleus

epizootic
: an outbreak of disease affecting large numbers of animals within a short time (equivalent to an epidemic relating to humans)

fox-adapted rabies	a strain of rabies virus serotype 1 to which the red fox is highly susceptible
frugivorous	fruit-eating
genotype	a group of organisms with similar genetic constitution
glycoprotein	a compound consisting of carbohydrate and protein. Club shaped glycoprotein molecules project from the surface of the rabies virus, and they are important in stimulating the host's immune response
host	living organism which supports the life of a parasitic organism eg a fox may be the host to the rabies virus
hydrophobia	literally a fear of water. A symptom of furious rabies in some humans
hypersensitivity	excessive sensitivity to external stimuli or foreign substances
immunity	the ability to resist disease
immunization	the administration of vaccine or hyperimmune serum (antibodies) to produce immunity to a disease
incubation period	the time between exposure to an infectious disease and the appearance of the first signs or symptoms
insectivorous	feeding on insects
intracerebral	within the brain
intradermal	(injection) delivered into the skin
intramuscular	(injection) delivered into muscle tissue
mucous membrane	a mucous secreting membrane which lines the body cavities or passages that are open to the external environment
myxomatosis	an infectious and usually fatal viral disease of rabbits
Negri bodies	red-staining area seen by microscopy in the cytoplasm of brain cells indicating rabies infection
oral vaccine	vaccine administered by mouth

pathogenicity	ability to cause disease
post-exposure prophylaxis	treatment designed to prevent disease given after contact with rabies virus
pre-exposure prophylaxis	treatment designed to prevent disease given before infection
primary vector (of rabies)	the main species responsible for carrying the rabies virus from one animal species to another
prodromai	relating to any symptoms which signal the impending onset of disease
rabies hyperimmune serum/globulin (RIG)	serum from an animal or human containing a large amount of rabies antibody, used to provide immediate (passive) immunization as part of post-exposure prophylaxis
rabies-enzootic country	a country where rabies is continuously present among animals, in contrast to an epizooric (qv)
rabies-susceptible animals	theoretically all warm blooded animals which may be infected with the rabies virus. Term usually refers to mammals most liable to be infected with the rabies virus
recombinant rabies vaccine	vaccine made by inserting nucleic acid sequences from a rabies virus into another virus (e.g. a poxvirus)
RNA	ribonucleic acid - genetic material present in all living cells. Unlike DNA it is single-stranded and has the sugar ribose instead of deoxyribuse and the base uracil instead of thymine
serology	a branch of science concerned with the reactions of blood sera, including the use of antibody tests
serotype	a closely related group of organisms, classified by means of serological tests
serum (fil sera)	fluid that remains after blood has been allowed to clot

sylvatic rabies	rabies infection maintained through a wildlife reservoir, as opposed to urban rabies which is maintained through the domestic and stray dog population
titre	(of antibody). A quantitative measure of antibody. (The highest dilution of serum at which antibody is detectable)
transmission	the passing of infection from one organism to another
vaccinia virus	a poxvirus originally used as a vaccine to protect against smallpox. It can be genetically engineered to produce other viral protein (e.g. rabies glycoprotein) for use as a vaccine
vector	an animal carrying an infection from one host to another
virulent	highly infective
virus	a micro-organism consisting of a DNA or RNA core surrounded by protein, which can only replicate in the cells of a host organism

Chapter 1

Introduction: the threat of rabies

The existence of rabies has been known for over 2000 years and its horrific symptoms followed by virtually inevitable death have made it notorious among diseases. It was known in classical Greece, where its link with dogs was understood. Rabies was documented in Britain as long ago as 1166.[1] The most important vectors in Britain were dogs, although other species were also infected, as occurred in an outbreak among deer in Richmond Park in 1886.[2]

How rabies was eradicated from Britain

Throughout the nineteenth century outbreaks of canine rabies in Britain led to human and animal deaths and thousands of dogs were slaughtered.[3] In 1874 a peak number of 74 human deaths was recorded by the Registrar-General.[4]

In the preceding years, Britain had witnessed an increase in state intervention, often enforced by statute, in many areas of life, not least in public health and preventive medicine. Pressure was brought to bear, by men such as Edwin Chadwick, urging government to take responsibility for the control of disease. Although there was considerable opposition to such centralized control of public health policy and activity, government took action to prevent further human deaths from rabies in the form of a series of Acts of Parliament.[5] These succeeded to varying degrees and culminated in the eradication of rabies from the British Isles.

Legislation in the form of a 'Bill to Prevent the Spreading of Canine Madness' was introduced in 1831, but proved limited in its impact; it was not until 1866 that the first effective anti-rabies legislation was passed. There followed several moves to control the disease including the Metropolitan Street Act of 1867 empowering the police to seize and destroy stray dogs, and making rabies a notifiable disease under the Contagious Diseases (Animals) Act in 1886. These Acts were followed by the Rabies Order of 1887 which gave local authorities powers to muzzle and control dogs and to destroy strays. Local control was then centralized to some degree with the passing of the Rabies City and Metropolitan Police Districts Order of 1889. The 1887 Order was inadequately enforced leading to a new order: the Rabies (Muzzling of Dogs) Order 1890. Although this latter Order achieved substantial successes, the public's dislike of muzzling led to the Order being revoked in 1892, resulting in an upsurge in cases, peaking in 1895 at 727 animal cases.[6] It was not until 1897 that import restrictions were imposed on dogs through the Rabies Order and Importation of Dogs Order.[7]

The dog import restrictions of 1897 set out that imported dogs must be licensed and quarantined in the owner's house for six months. Since this system was abused and proved impractical to regulate, the Order was revoked by the 1901 Order, which retained the requirement of a licence for dogs landed in Britain except for those from Ireland, the Channel Islands and the Isle of Man. These licensed dogs had to be kept in isolation for six months on premises under the control of a veterinary surgeon and completely separate from their owners. Foreign dogs on board vessels in harbour had to be securely confined. These Acts and Orders led to the eradication of rabies from Britain for the first time in 1902. Cats, which are subject to much less legislation than dogs, were only included in the restrictions in 1928 with the Importation of Dogs and Cats Order, despite their similar susceptibility to rabies.

Quarantine in Britain

For a brief time, the quarantine period was reduced to four months in 1914, though this was later restored to six months. The country remained rabies-free until 1918, when Britain was re-infected with rabies following the smuggling of animals, probably by servicemen returning from the Continent. The disease spread rapidly through the south of England and South Wales and before it was again eradicated in 1922, 358 people were known to have been bitten by rabid or suspected rabid animals. Between 1918 and 1922 there were confirmed cases in 312 dogs, eight cattle, two sheep, three pigs and three horses.

It was possible to eradicate rabies from Britain at this time because the disease was predominantly carried by dogs in urban areas. Unlike today's European epizootic (an endemic amongst animals), it was not sustained through a reservoir of infection in the fox population. It is thought that at some time in the past rabies may have occurred in wildlife in Britain and then died out naturally, as has been seen in some other European countries. In Switzerland fox rabies was predominant until around 1929, but was then absent until 1967 when the virus was re-introduced by infected foxes crossing the German border.[2]

For Britain to regain its rabies-free status, as it did in 1922, quarantine regulations had to be strengthened, muzzle and leash restrictions introduced and strays destroyed. No rabid animal was free in Britain until 1969 and 1970 when two dogs developed rabies after release from quarantine.

On 26 July 1969 a collie imported from India died of rabies in quarantine. It had reportedly been involved in a fight with a stray dog in India one month before importation. On 18 October that year another dog, from the same kennels as the collie, died of rabies ten days after its release from quarantine. This was the first animal to die of rabies outside quarantine or other confined premises since 1922. It had either contracted rabies before importation, in which case it was one of the rare cases with an incubation period longer than six months, or it had become infected by indirect contact with another dog during its period of quarantine.

Upon discovery that the rabid dog had been exercised over a wide area near Camberley, Surrey, action was taken to prevent the spread of rabies by restricting the movement of dogs housed in the immediate area. The public was asked to help identify any contacts that the dog may have had and, as a precaution, susceptible wildlife in the surrounding area was poisoned or shot.

There followed on 13 November 1969 a third dog in the same kennels which developed symptoms. The dog was destroyed and rabies was confirmed by laboratory tests. An inquiry set up in October 1969 concluded that there was a strong possibility that at least one of the three dogs had contracted rabies in quarantine, but whether by direct or indirect contact was unknown.

In 1970 a fourth dog, brought to Britain from Pakistan in May 1969, developed rabies and died in Newmarket three months after its release from quarantine. In the light of evidence of a significant amount of smuggling taking place, it was feared that the dog imported from Pakistan may have contracted rabies *after* leaving quarantine, although no evidence was advanced to support this hypothesis.[8]

Following these incidents the Committee of Inquiry on Rabies was appointed in April 1970 under the chairmanship of Ronald Waterhouse QC to review control procedures. Meanwhile, quarantine was extended to eight months (in December 1969) and then to 12 months after the Newmarket incident while the committee was deliberating. In September 1970 it was restored to six months following the findings of the Waterhouse Committee, which was to report in 1971. Following the recommendation of the Waterhouse Committee, all dogs and cats are now given prophylactic vaccination on entering quarantine. Britain has remained free of reported disease ever since, and not one of nearly 200 000 cats and dogs vaccinated in quarantine has succumbed to rabies after release from quarantine.

Rabies in Europe

Historically rabies has been widespread in Europe among various species. In France, where the disease was enzootic, bites from wolves led to the deaths of many people. In 1851, during the course of a single day in Hue-Au-Gal, one rabid wolf bit 46 persons and 82 head of cattle.[9]

At the beginning of this century dog rabies disappeared from Western European countries, but by the end of the Second World War 'sylvatic' rabies, where the disease is maintained through a wildlife reservoir, had invaded most of eastern and central Europe, eventually reaching Switzerland, Belgium, the east of France and the north of Italy. Mainland Norway, Sweden and Finland, the British Isles, Ireland, Spain, Portugal and Greece remained rabies-free. The outbreak, carried by foxes, is thought to have originated in 1939–40 at the Russian-Polish border, before advancing westwards across Europe after the Second World War. Since 1939 it has spread some 1400 kilometres westward.[10] The Second World War may have been a contributory factor to its spread by the movement of armies which brought destruction of ecosystems and displaced fox populations.[11]

Rabid foxes moved from Poland to East Germany in 1948 and across the German plain until, by 1950, West Germany was affected with the disease moving northwards through Schleswig-Holstein to Denmark. Denmark is now free of terrestrial rabies, but has encountered problems with rabid foxes entering from Germany and Schleswig-Holstein. Rabies reached France from Germany in 1968. By 1984 a quarter of the country had been affected. Wildlife rabies was established in the northernmost part of Italy, crossing the Alpine passes from Austria and Switzerland, but this outbreak died out in 1969. A second wave entered Italy in September 1978 and in 1994 rabies was reported in the Po Valley.[12]

Recently, the advance of the epizootic, which had previously progressed at between 20 and 60 kilometres a year, appears to have stopped. No definitive cause has been found for this:[10] there were no geographical barriers, there was no lack of susceptible foxes and the wave-front was not halted by the reduction of fox numbers or by oral vaccination.

Rabies outside Europe

Dog rabies remains highly prevalent in most of the countries of Africa, Asia and Latin America, where millions of people are at risk of infection with the disease posing a major threat to public health. In India every year some 25 000 people are reported to die from rabies and three million are treated for exposure.[13,14]

Pasteur's experiments

The first rabies vaccine was developed by Louis Pasteur in 1885. Uncharacteristically for his time, he believed that rabies did not occur

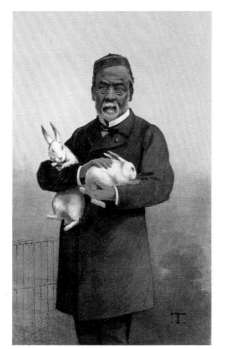

spontaneously in dogs but that each case was caused by another. The link between being bitten and infection pointed to saliva as a source of the infective organism, and Pasteur carried out a series of experiments to investigate, even collecting saliva from rabid dogs for this purpose, at great personal risk. Pasteur and his co-workers showed that the rabies virus was consistently present in the central nervous system of animals dying of the disease.

Pasteur had already succeeded in producing attenuated (weakened) strains of chicken cholera and anthrax, which were used to vaccinate animals against these diseases, and he applied similar principles to rabies. He passed the virus repeatedly through rabbits, which do not maintain the virus in the wild, altering and attenuating it (though this has also been attributed to Galtier in 1899). By attenuating the virus the disease's incubation period was simultaneously shortened to a fixed period of five to eight days, when introduced intracerebrally into dogs.

Louis Pasteur with rabbits (1822 – 95)

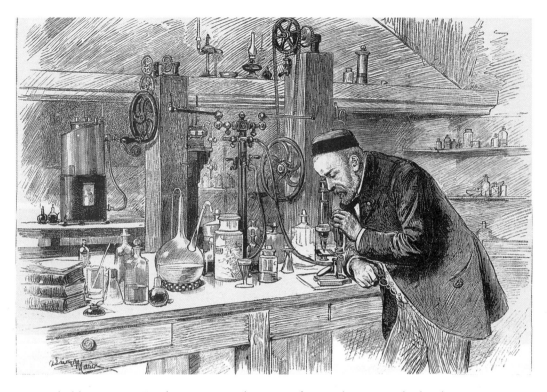

Pasteur in his laboratory   Fixed or attenuated strains of virus show a marked reduction in infectivity when inoculated subcutaneously into the original hosts but infectivity is not entirely eliminated and may vary with the strain of virus, the dosage and host to which it is administered; its virulence is often increased when inoculated intracerebrally.

Pasteur prepared a vaccine by taking spinal cords from rabbits that had died from infection with fixed virus seven days earlier. The cords were suspended in flasks and dried over caustic potash. The infectivity of the virus diminished the longer the cords were dried. In tests, dogs were inoculated with suspensions of cords that had been dried for shorter and shorter periods, thus containing progressively more of the weakened live virus. The dogs eventually became resistant to infection, even when fully virulent virus was inoculated intracerebrally.

The first use of the vaccine on a human was the case of a boy bitten by a rabid dog in 1885. Joseph Meister had been badly bitten when brought to Pasteur. Were the treatment to go wrong, Pasteur would face severe criticism, and so he consulted the opinions of two doctors. All agreed that untreated the boy would develop rabies and die and Pasteur wrote 'that although more than 200 vaccinated dogs had resisted challenge ... it was not without great anxiety and doubts that we decided that the child would be vaccinated'. Joseph Meister was injected daily with progressively more potent doses of Pasteur's preparation of rabbit cords. Meister did not develop rabies and survived the treatment, living on to be employed as a doorman at the Pasteur Institute in Paris. Although this success gained Pasteur widespread public acclaim, brain tissue vaccines have side-effects which can include death.

Since Pasteur's breakthrough, there have been considerable advances in the development of human anti-rabies vaccines, bringing improvements in both safety and efficacy. With prompt treatment, deaths from rabies or the side-effects of vaccines are rare. A number of different virus strains and cell lines are now used to produce vaccines for human use around the world (Appendices I and II). Several highly effective and safe vaccines are available, but there are considerable differences in cost. The only vaccine licensed for human use in Britain (human diploid cell vaccine), costs more than double the French purified vero cell (green monkey kidney cell line) vaccine (PVRV) and the German purified chick embryo cell vaccine (PCEC). There appears to be no reason why these French and German vaccines should not be licensed for use in Britain.

Table 1 Classification of rabies and rabies-related Lyssaviruses. Their sources and geographic distribution

Virus name serotype	Source(s) of virus in nature	Known geographic distribution
Rabies 1	dog, cat, bat, human; wild carnivores, e.g. red, grey, bat-eared fox, skunk, raccoon, jackal, mongoose	worldwide except Australia, New Zealand, Antarctica, parts of Scandinavia, United Kingdom, Japan, Hawaii and some other islands
Lagos bat 2	frugivorous bat, cat, dog	Nigeria, Ethiopia, Senegal, Central African Republic, Zimbabwe, South Africa
a Mokola 3	shrew, cat, dog, rodent, human	Nigeria, Ethiopia, Cameroon, Central African Republic, Zimbabwe, South Africa
a Duvenhage 4	insectivorous bat, human	Zimbabwe, South Africa
EBL subtype 1 unclassified; probably genotype 5	insectivorous bat (chiefly serotines), human	Germany, Poland, Ukraine, Netherlands, Denmark, France, Spain
EBL subtype 2 unclassified; probably genotype 6	insectivorous bat (Myotis spp.), human	Netherlands, Switzerland, Finland

a Although the rabies-related Mokola and Duvenhage viruses rarely infect man, each has caused a human death.[15] The patient with Duvenhage virus had clinical features identical to furious rabies[16, 17]

The natural history of rabies

Rabies, from *'rabere'* in Latin, meaning 'to rave', is a member of the large genus Lyssavirus (lyssa meaning 'rage' in Greek) within the large family known as the Rhabdoviridae (rod-shaped). Lyssaviruses also include the rabies-related viruses listed in Table 1. The widespread rabies 'street virus' is of serotype 1, and causes the vast majority of rabies-like disease. Minor differences in strains of rabies virus isolated from different vector species and in different geographical areas can now be distinguished by monoclonal antibody techniques and by nucleotide sequencing.

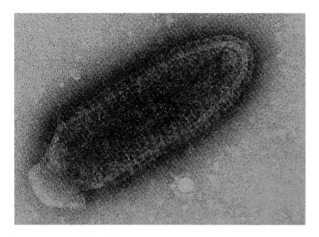

Electronmicrograph of rabies virus

The rabies-related viruses are a group of five Lyssaviruses antigenically similar to rabies. They are classified thus: serotype 2 (Lagos bat), serotype 3 (Mokola), serotype 4 (Duvenhage) and the European bat Lyssaviruses (EBL) subtype 1 (EBL1) and subtype 2 (EBL2) (the nomenclature of classification will be changed from serotype to genotype with EBL 1 and EBL 2 classified as genotypes 5 and 6 respectively). Mokola and Duvenhage viruses have only been found in Africa. All these viruses except Lagos bat virus have been known to cause death in humans. Rabies-related virus infections, ie infections caused by serotypes other than serotype 1, are very rarely identified.

Rabies in animals

All warm-blooded animals are susceptible to rabies virus infection, but susceptibility varies widely between different species. The most highly susceptible experimentally are foxes, coyotes, jackals, wolves, kangaroo rats, cotton rats and common field voles.[18] Dogs, although experimentally only moderately susceptible, are the main source of the infection in humans.

Rabies strains sometimes show species adaptation and this may be of particular significance within Europe. The fox-adapted rabies strain prevalent throughout Western Europe is said to be poorly transmissible within other species and it has never been documented that dogs or cats have spread fox-adapted rabies virus into new, previously rabies-free areas. This concept is of significance for UK quarantine because if correct, it means that dogs and cats imported from the EU are very unlikely to transmit rabies virus into UK wildlife, but the debate continues.

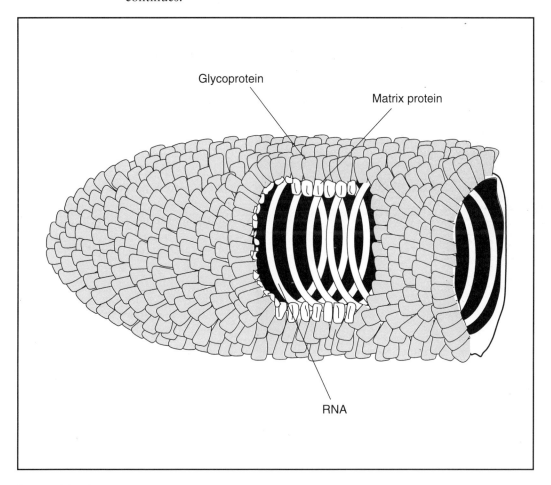

Structure of the rabies virus

Clinical signs in animals

Normally, domestic pets are friendly, are not easily disturbed, look healthy and exhibit a predictable behavioural pattern. Wild animals also exhibit characteristic behavioural patterns – normally they are afraid of man and in a free environment they usually prefer to slip away unseen and to avoid contact. Exceptions to this retiring behaviour may occur: normally shy wild animals may become semi-tame as a result of protection and feeding, especially in parks and campsites, where, in close contact with man, their normal character may be abandoned as they learn to take food from holidaymakers.

Rabid animals do not behave normally. The signs of disease are quite variable and duration of illness may range from less than one day to a week or more; death often intervenes two to seven days after onset of illness. Clinical disease may take either the 'dumb' form (also known as 'paralytic' rabies) or the 'furious' form or most often a combination of the two. In dumb rabies the symptoms are more tranquil. Hypersensitivity, where the animal reacts excessively to stimuli such as noise or being touched, is not readily apparent though it may occur as a minor and transient manifestation. The first changes seen in a normal, healthy animal are somewhat benign: the animal is lethargic, appears unhealthy with some slight inco-ordination. This condition may remain stable for about 12 hours then deteriorate rapidly and loss of the swallowing reflex may be observed, though dogs do not exhibit the fear of water (hydrophobia) common in humans, and the animal may die without other signs.

In the first 'prodromal' stage of furious rabies, the pet animal appears unusually alert and responsive and the owner may interpret this as the pet being particularly well. This slight behavioural change would not be readily recognized in a wild animal. The abnormally alert pet, however, soon shows discomfort and unease. Cats in particular show an uneasy facial expression and frequently mew, repeatedly extend and retract their claws and exhibit a restless dancing movement of the front feet.

Dog with furious rabies. (Reproduced by permission of the World Health Organization ©)

They may respond to prodding, showing impatience and intolerance of minor irritations.

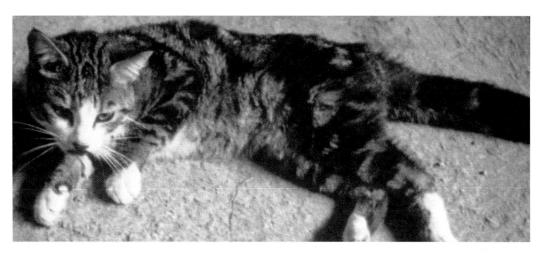

Cat with rabies

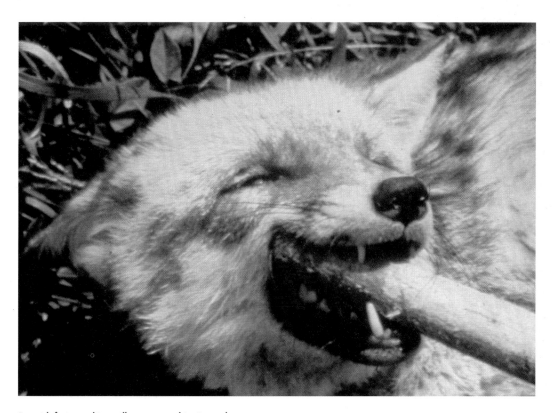

Fox with furious rabies: will snap at anything in reach

Rabid wild animals show similar signs of sensitivity and discomfort and may bite at a source of irritation as hypersensitivity to external irritation increases; they will snap at anything within reach and in biting they may hold tenaciously, making them particularly dangerous vectors of the virus. Irritation at the site of virus inoculation (usually a bite) may result in their constant licking and chewing of the infected area. Compulsive seizures may then develop; these may become almost continuous until death, usually from respiratory arrest. Ascending paralysis is commonly seen in wild as well as domestic animals.

Confusion and disorientation are consistent signs of rabies in both domestic and wild animals. Wild animals may lose their normal caution and wander into farmyards, suburbs and campsites; such aberrant behaviour is common. Early signs in dogs last two to five days and are followed by dumb rabies in 75% of cases, or furious rabies in the remainder. Paralysis and death occur in both dumb and furious forms of the disease four to eight days after the onset of symptoms. However, virus may be present in the saliva of rabid animals for many days before clinical signs appear and it may be steadily or intermittently secreted until just before death. Cats usually develop furious rabies and are especially dangerous to man since, as lap animals, they are more likely to strike at the face and neck.

Rabies in man

The most common means of transmitting rabies virus is via the bite of a diseased animal depositing the virus in the tissues. The virus cannot penetrate unbroken skin, but it can enter the body across intact mucous membranes, such as the lining of the nose and mouth, or the conjunctiva of the eye. Transmission from person to person has never been reliably documented, except in the case of corneal transplants (the transparent surface of the front of the eyeball) from donors who have died from unsuspected rabies infection.[11] Other diseases can be transmitted in this way including cryptococcosis and Creutzfeldt-Jakob disease.

More rarely, rabies infection may occur through inhalation, vaccination and transplant. Inhalation of airborne rabies virus may be a route of infection for animals such as bats, but is extremely rare in humans.[11] Post-vaccinal rabies (*rage de laboratoire*) is caused by inoculation with anti-rabies vaccine in which an attenuated virus has reverted to virulence or the virus has not been properly inactivated. The virus used in some veterinary vaccines and in older types of human vaccine used in some developing countries was inactivated by phenol or

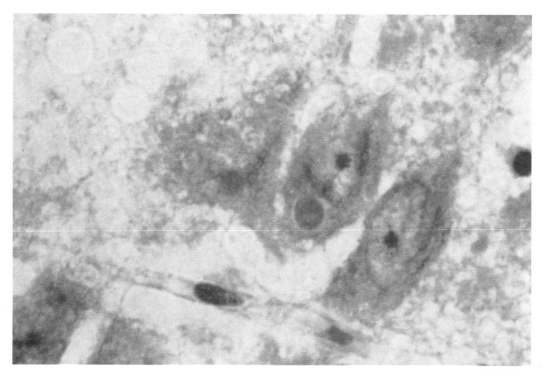

Diagnosis of rabies encephalitis was originally made by finding Negri bodies (red-staining areas) in the cytoplasm of neurones in the brain

formaldehyde, but these treatments have been known on rare occasions to fail. In many modern human vaccines, virus is inactivated by ß-propiolactone, which removes its infectivity more reliably.

The time between exposure to the virus and the onset of symptoms varies widely, with a range of four days to many years.[11] This incubation period may depend upon the site that the virus enters the body (bites on or near the head tend to reach the central nervous system faster) the severity of the bite, the age of the victim (children tend to develop rabies more quickly, but this may be due to children being bitten more severely or nearer the head) or to the virulence of the virus strain. During the incubation period the virus may or may not replicate in the tissues before it reaches a peripheral nerve through which it travels to the spinal cord and then to the brain. In over 60% of cases the incubation period for humans lies between 20 and 90 days. Once clinical symptoms of rabies appear, there is no known cure and the victim is virtually certain to die an agonizing and terrifying death.

The clinical course in humans

From the onset of symptoms of clinical rabies, death ensues in an average of three to seven days in untreated cases. It has been known for people to survive rabies encephalitis, but this is extremely rare. Among these few survivors, one patient was left with severe neurological complications.[19] The hopeless outlook for anyone developing symptoms of rabies adds to the terror of the disease.

The prodromal stage may be characterized by influenza-like symptoms: fever, loss of appetite, headache, other aches and pains, weakness and tiredness. Sometimes the first symptoms are itching or abnormal sensation, such as burning or stabbing pain, at the site of the bite. The victim may also suffer from anxiety, restlessness, depression, a feeling of tension, insomnia, lack of concentration, and even in those unaware of the possible diagnosis of rabies, a sense of foreboding. This stage is associated with the virus's invasion of the central nervous system.

The second stage may be characterized by either furious rabies, the more common form in humans, or paralytic rabies. With furious rabies the victim may display excitement, aggression, spasms, frothing at the mouth, difficulty in swallowing, hallucination followed by lucid moments and distressing spasms involving the inspiratory muscles. One of the most notorious symptoms is hydrophobia (literally a dread of

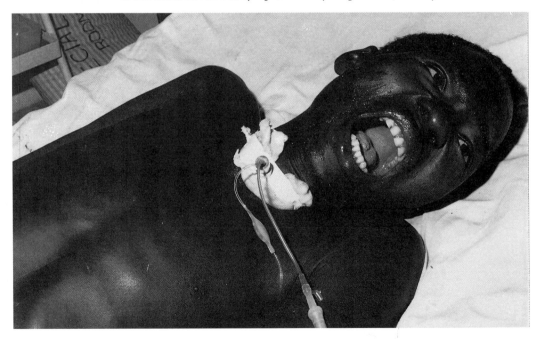

Nigerian man with furious rabies

water), precipitated by attempts to drink. When a glass of water is brought to the mouth, the victim may take a series of jerky inspirations, his head jolts uncontrollably backwards and his arms are thrown upward, spilling the liquid. As the disease progresses, the mere mention or sight of water is enough to bring on this response. The mechanism of hydrophobia is not completely understood, but a hypothesis has been advanced by Warrell, Davidson, Pope et al.[20] In rabies the muscles of the pharynx, which control swallowing, are weakened allowing water to come into contact with the entrance of the larynx and the back of the nose. This triggers coughing and other reflexes which cause a sharp indrawing of breath characteristic of the spasms of hydrophobia. The associated terror is thought to be a result of the infection and inflammation of those areas of the brain which are responsible for such emotions as fear and aggression. Death may result from generalized convulsions or through a steady deterioration of mental function over several days into coma. Although the exact cause of death is usually unknown, it is believed that the brain-stem encephalitis (inflammation of the brain) destroys control of vital functions leading to respiratory and cardiac arrest.[11]

Paralytic rabies is less common in humans (though the more common form in most animals) and is harder to diagnose than the furious form. This is particularly the case in rural areas of developing countries where it may be mistaken for poliomyelitis or Guillain-Barré syndrome. At least five corneas have been unwittingly transplanted from donors with paralytic rabies. Paralytic rabies is characteristic of infection by fixed virus rabies acquired from vaccination (rage de laboratoire) and infection by vampire bats. Paralysis usually starts in the bitten area and ascends progressively. Another symptom is 'fasciculation', the trembling contraction of certain muscle fibres with an appearance rather like shivering. Hydrophobia is rare in patients with paralytic rabies but during the last stages of the disease, and just before coma, the distinction between dumb rabies and the furious forms may be less clear; patients with dumb rabies may exhibit hydrophobic reactions at this stage. Death from furious rabies is much quicker than from the paralytic form of the disease. In the latter, death usually follows paralysis of the breathing and swallowing muscles but patients may survive for up to 30 days even without intensive care.[11]

Due to the wide availability of post-exposure treatment, human deaths from rabies are very rare in the west. For this reason, and also the non-specific symptoms of the prodromal phase, diagnosis is difficult. In the United States, three human rabies cases since 1985 have only been diagnosed a month after death.[21]

The following case history appears courtesy of Professor D A Warrell.

A 23-year-old English woman died of rabies in England on 24 August 1981. On 17 June, whilst on holiday in a village in Himachal Pradesh in the Himalayan foothills 500 kilometres from Delhi, she was bitten on the leg by a neighbour's pet dog. Her husband cleaned the wound, using whisky as an antiseptic. They went immediately to a nearby village to consult the local doctor, who cleaned the wound with iodine and dressed it with antiseptic powder. They asked for a tetanus injection, but were told that none was available in that valley. The doctor gave the patient vitamins, antibiotic capsules, and a homeopathic remedy. He asked them if the dog was mad, but they denied this, saying that it was a pet dog defending its territory. They returned to the doctor four times to have the wound dressed, but after a week the patient decided to continue this unaided.

They returned to England one month after the bite and, two days later (20 July), went to their local hospital. The patient explained to a nursing sister in the casualty department that the bite on her leg, still unhealed, had been inflicted by a dog in India. A swab was taken for bacterial culture and the wound scraped and then dressed each day for five days. There was such improvement that the couple went off hop-picking in Kent.

About two months after the bite, the patient experienced her first prodromal symptoms of rabies. Tiredness after an all-night party persisted for three days and she noticed aching and shooting pains in the waist and small of her back. She had missed two monthly periods and wondered if she were pregnant. She became anxious and depressed and that night (18 August) seemed to catch her breath when she tried to drink. Next day she consulted her general practitioner. He thought that her symptoms were related to anxiety about the suspected pregnancy. It became impossible for her to drink more than small sips of liquid. When she rode on her husband's motorbike the wind made her catch her breath and that night she could not bear the feeling of her hair against her face. Frequently she sat up in bed, apparently terrified. The next day her legs felt heavy, painful and so tender that she could not bear to have the cat sitting on her lap. She developed a stomach upset. That night she was confused, hallucinated, and incontinent of urine and was intermittently hallucinating and screaming with terror. Her general practitioner's partner was persuaded to give her an injection of tranquillizer. He considered that she was suffering from hysteria and arranged for her to be visited at home by two psychiatric social workers. By the evening she was so wild and agitated that her husband felt he could not cope with her alone, so he took her to her mother's house. Just before midnight she awoke in a terrified state and collapsed on the way to the lavatory. The general practitioner on duty again reassured them over the telephone that she was suffering from a mental condition and that nothing need be done. She continued in a state of terror, hallucination and pain throughout the night. Early next morning her pulse seemed to stop and an ambulance was summoned by emergency call. While she was being carried out of the house she had a cardiac arrest from which she was resuscitated. She was taken to the Intensive Care unit of the local hospital, where she died less than 48 hours later, without recovering consciousness. Rabies infection was confirmed.[22]

This case illustrates the importance for travellers to be aware of the dangers in rabies-endemic areas. Countries of particularly high risk are those where medical attention, particularly in rural areas, is limited, and those which are affected by dog rabies, the major source of human exposure. Travel to such countries has become increasingly common in recent years and general practitioners and travel agents should be provided with information for advising travellers. In its general guidance on rabies, the Department of Health advises doctors on alerting travellers going abroad, but there is a lack of up-to-date details regarding which countries are affected.[18] Similarly the Department of Health's leaflet for the public *Health advice for travellers anywhere in the world* omits any comprehensive list of those countries with endemic rabies.

Pre-exposure vaccination is safe and effective and should be considered by anyone spending time in rural areas of rabies-enzootic countries, or those more than a day's journey from a source of post-exposure treatment.[23] Advice on avoiding contact with animals should also be given. Anyone bitten by a suspect animal should seek medical attention immediately and should accept nothing less than:

• thorough cleaning of the wound

• post-exposure vaccination

• hyperimmune serum.

If any one of these treatments is unavailable or inadequate, travellers should consider cutting short their holiday in order to return home for immediate treatment.

Public attitudes to rabies, quarantine and change

In spite of the rarity of such cases of human rabies and the availability of safe and effective vaccines in the developed world, the British public continues to perceive rabies as a terrifying disease to be kept out of Britain at all costs. There are several reasons for this attitude. Britain's rabies-free status is seen as a major advantage, in which the nation may take pride. Quarantine regulations are equated with this freedom from rabies; any significant change to these is seen as a direct threat to that much prized status. In countries such as France, affected by enzootic rabies, there is an entirely different attitude to the disease.

Effective government campaigns contribute to the British fear of rabies; propaganda has included leaflets, educational films, radio broadcasts and posters, declaring 'Bringing it in is MADNESS'. In its publication *Rabies prevention and control*, MAFF stated 'The Government regard the active support of the public as a vital part of the defences against rabies' and the Government does indeed receive such support from the public.[24] In one anecdotal case, vigilant shoppers in Oxford Street, London, spotted a dog in a car with German number plates and alerted the Ministry. It transpired that the dog had been smuggled into the country and was therefore a potential rabies threat.

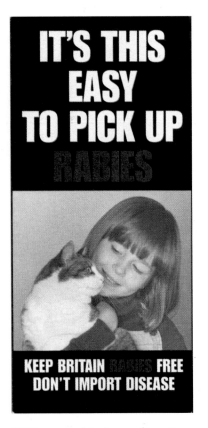

MAFF's warning of the dangers of importing rabies into Britain

Within Europe, most nations affected by rabies live with the disease in their wildlife and accept it. It may be difficult for other member states of the EU to appreciate the depth of feeling provoked by changes or proposed changes to quarantine regulations. Persuading the British public that the threat from rabies is less serious than in previous decades and that different methods of control could be equally effective – claims which are open to question – is likely to prove difficult.

Chapter 2

Current rabies legislation

Until July 1994, there was no distinction between pets and commercially traded animals in legislation governing their import; all dogs, cats and other rabies susceptible animals (except farm stock and equines) had to enter rabies quarantine. Following the creation of the single European market, commercially traded cats and dogs, whose movement was hampered by quarantine, have been allowed to enter Britain under the requirements of the Balai Directive (Council Directive 92/65/EEC of 13 July 1992). This directive states that certain commercially traded animals should be allowed into the UK without having to spend six months in quarantine on import. MAFF maintains that the priority of current policy remains the safeguarding of Britain from rabies.[24]

The importation into Britain of domestic pets is governed by the Rabies (Importation of Dogs, Cats and Other Mammals) Order 1974 as amended in 1994. Pets are defined as any dog, cat or other mammal which has not been permanently kept on the premises in which it was born. Guide dogs, guard dogs, sniffer dogs and any similar working animals are therefore classified as pets. This legislation does not include farm stock and some other herbivores, such as horses and other equines, which, while susceptible to rabies, are not considered significant vectors of the disease by MAFF. However, if the animals in this group have been in contact with animals that are subject to quarantine regulations, they too will be subject to control under the Order. They are also subject to other animal health import controls which provide safeguards against rabies.

All circus animals which are rabies susceptible such as lions and tigers, must be quarantined. However, very few circus troupes bring their animals into Britain. Those choosing to do so generally quarantine their animals in Britain over the winter. Circuses from abroad generally hire British animals for their shows in this country.

The main provisions of the Rabies (Importation of Dogs, Cats and Other Mammals) Order 1974 (as amended) are as follows.[24]

- The landing in Great Britain of a pet animal brought from outside Britain is prohibited except in accordance with the terms of a licence issued in advance (Article 4 (1) and (3)).

- The prohibition does not apply to pet animals brought from Northern Ireland, the Channel Islands, the Republic of Ireland or the Isle of Man, unless the animals have been brought to those countries from elsewhere and have not undergone at least six months quarantine before being landed in Great Britain (Article 4 (2)).

- Licensed landings are permitted only at ports and airports authorised in Schedule 2 (as amended) to the Order unless the vessel or aircraft has been diverted in the interests of safety, or in other exceptional circumstances (Article 4(5)).

- Any pet animal taken to a place outside the British Isles and brought back, whether or not it landed in that place, or an animal which, while outside Great Britain has had contact with an animal to which importation controls apply, is an imported pet animal for the purposes of the Order (Article 4 (8) (a) and (b)).

- Pet animals imported under licence must be detained in quarantine for at least 6 months at the owners' expense (Articles 5 (1)–(4)). Quarantine may be extended in the case of a rabies outbreak at quarantine premises (Article 5 (5))*.

- Dogs and cats in quarantine must be vaccinated against rabies (Article 6 (1)), with exemption provision where the dog or cat has been imported for research purposes with which vaccination might interfere (Article 6(2)).

- Pet animals imported in accordance with a licence must be taken from the port of entry to quarantine premises by an authorised carrying agent (Article 7).

- An animal passing through Great Britain must remain within the confines of the port or airport while awaiting trans-shipment, and may only be moved within the port or airport by an authorised carrying agent. It must be exported from the port or airport within 48 hours, and if remaining there for more than four hours it must be retained in authorised holding premises until re-embarkation (Article 8).

- Pet animals from abroad on board vessels in harbour in Great Britain must be restrained and securely confined in a totally enclosed part of the vessel, prevented from contact with any other animals, and in no circumstances permitted to land (except in accordance with an importation licence) (Article 12).

- Animals in relation to which there are contraventions of, or failure to comply with provisions of the Order may be seized and, if appropriate, destroyed (Articles 12, 13 and 14).

  Vampire bats must be kept in quarantine conditions for life, ie in isolation from other species (this could be arranged in a zoo), as they are thought to be capable of carrying the virus throughout their lives and passing it on to their offspring

Import of commercially traded animals from the EU[25]

A commercially traded cat or dog is one imported as the subject of a commercial transaction. The main requirements for cats and dogs imported to Britain for purposes of commercial trading following the July 1994 implementation of the Balai Directive, are that the animal must:

- have no signs of contagious disease on dispatch

- be fitted with a microchip implant to enable identification, accompanied by a reader able to read the implanted microchip

- be certified never to have left the registered premises on which it was born (except for attending a veterinary practice for treatment under restraint)

- have no contact with wild animals

- have been vaccinated against rabies (and dogs additionally against distemper)

- have been blood tested to show a minimum antibody level of 0.5 IU for rabies

- be accompanied by health and vaccination certificates signed by an Official Veterinary Surgeon.

An Official Veterinary Surgeon is a veterinarian designated by the competent central authority of the EU member state. The qualifications necessary to be considered a veterinarian within the EU were laid down in EU Directive 78/1026/EEC in 1978. The local British Divisional Veterinary Officer (DVO) must be notified in advance of the animal's arrival and it will be examined at its destination (i.e. once inside the country rather than at the border) within 48 hours of its arrival. The animal must then not be moved from the premises of destination for ten days while the results of blood tests, if considered necessary, are awaited. The serological tests must be carried out in accordance with the World

Health Organization's (WHO) specifications. If the animal fails to fulfil these requirements, it will be subject to six months quarantine.[25] These new regulations do not apply to pets or rabies susceptible animals moving between the UK and Ireland, the Channel Islands or the Isle of Man.

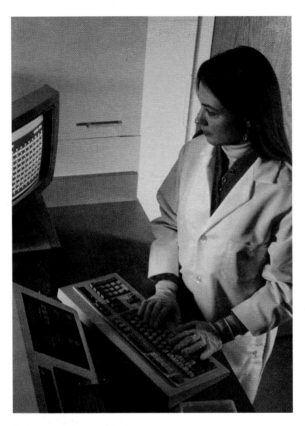

Technician carrying out blood tests

Offences under the Rabies (Importation of Dogs, Cats and other Mammals) Order 1974 can be dealt with either under summary proceedings, where the maximum penalty is a fine of £5000; or by an indictment (where there is evidence of deliberate intent to evade the provisions) where the maximum penalty is an unlimited fine and/or up to one year's imprisonment. In addition, the animal may be destroyed at the discretion of the enforcing authority.

It is against British law to vaccinate 'native' animals against rabies in the UK apart from those being exported or on entry to quarantine. The reasons given by MAFF are that it would be wasteful without providing a real safeguard; it would undermine confidence in the Government's policy of import control and quarantine and it would create a false climate of security which might encourage smuggling.[24]

Responsibilities for preventing rabies in the UK

Local authorities (normally at County level in England and Wales, Regional and Island Councils in Scotland) are the enforcement authorities, through their animals health inspectors, designated under the Animal Health Act 1981. The police and MAFF's inspectors appointed under the Animal Health Act 1981 also have enforcement powers.

In the course of normal customs surveillance, port and airport officials look not only for contraband substances such as narcotics but also for illegal landings of animals. However, following the lifting of European Union border barriers in January 1993, citizens of member states may now pass through a 'blue channel' free from customs checks, although spot checks may still be made and passports inspected.

Table 2 Responsibilities for preventing rabies in the UK

Department	Area of responsibility
Ministry of Agriculture, Fisheries and Food Scottish Office Agriculture and Fisheries Department Welsh Office Agriculture Department	central responsibility for campaign against rabies
Ministry of Agriculture, Fisheries and Food	operational control in case of a rabies outbreak
Customs and Excise	enforcement of import controls at the ports and airports (this includes the Channel Tunnel)
Department of Health	rabies in humans: prophylactic pre- and post-exposure vaccination
Department of the Environment	nature conservation; local implications
Home Office	cruelty against domestic and captive animals; police implications; penalties
Scottish Office	the special interests of Scotland
Welsh Office	the special interests of Wales

Shipping and airline companies are required to ensure that pet animals are not embarked without a boarding document confirming that an import licence has been granted. Airlines must also ensure that animals do not travel other than as 'manifested' freight (i.e. as cargo rather than baggage) in an approved container in the freight compartment, and that each container is properly labelled with an official rabies control transit label. Cargo, unlike baggage, must be accompanied by an airway bill which alerts Customs to its presence. No animals will be allowed to be taken on to trains travelling through the Channel Tunnel.

All authorized ports of entry are required to provide approved, secure holding facilities for the temporary retention of animals being trans-shipped and imported animals whose transport to approved quarantine premises is, for any reason, delayed. The capacity of each holding facility is required to be adequate to meet the throughput.

The Government keeps in contact with the appropriate authorities in Northern Ireland, the Republic of Ireland, the Channel Islands and the Isle of Man to ensure compatibility of legislation and regulations and to co-ordinate defences with the aim of keeping rabies out of the British Isles.

Chapter 3

Patterns of rabies around the world

Rabies is distributed very unevenly across the world, occurring in separate cycles within a few species of mammals in different geographical areas. As with many diseases, islands and peninsulae may remain free of rabies for extended periods. The way in which any virus spreads depends on the hosts available and those hosts' susceptibility to that virus; each strain of rabies virus is adapted to its host species, although infection can spill over to other mammals including man.

Worldwide prevalence of rabies

Calculating the incidence of rabies in both humans and animals is difficult. Its accurate diagnosis depends on the availability of diagnostic laboratories. While these are available in the developed world, there are few in developing countries. In the latter, most human and animal cases are diagnosed on clinical grounds only (i.e. from symptoms and clinical outcome, not laboratory tests), which are less reliable. Under-reporting of rabies cases may also occur.

In Europe and North America, although diagnostic facilities are usually available to ensure more accurate statistics for human rabies, the problem of detecting rabies cases among wildlife remains. Despite the World Health Organization's monitoring, it is impossible to estimate accurately how many rabid foxes there are in Europe. It has been suggested that for each fox diagnosed, eight or nine others may die undetected in underground burrows. The occurrence of rabies in fox cubs in the den is not accounted for, but could be frequent.[26]

There is no generally accepted method for accurately estimating fox numbers, and diagnosis of rabies in foxes relies on testing those that have been killed by hunters or found sick or dead. In France it is thought that changes in the prevalence of rabies in foxes can best be monitored by changes in the incidence of disease among domestic animals, among which cases are far easier to survey and diagnose.[11] While they may not be accurate in absolute numbers, the statistics are useful in indicating change.

As the incidence of fox rabies fluctuates through the year, comparison must be made of the same periods of the year over a number of years. For instance, it is thought that cases of fox rabies escalate in the late winter during the mating season when the contact rate increases.[12] It is with these provisos that statistics on the prevalence of rabies should be viewed.

Control of rabies around the world

The advance of rabies, as with many diseases, is aided by political instability. Following the break-up of the former Soviet Union and the consequent collapse of many public health measures several diseases, such as poliomyelitis, have re-emerged.[27] The growth of canine populations which accompanies the increases in human populations in many parts of the developing world hampers the population control of stray dogs and only nations with considerable resources for the task have succeeded.

Worldwide it is estimated that 94% of all rabies deaths are due to canine rabies. Vaccination of dogs in sufficient numbers has been shown to bring rabies under control in many of the countries where canine rabies is the predominant form of the disease. However, to be effective in preventing the wider spread of the disease at least 75% of the dogs must be reached.[28] In those Asian countries where vaccination of dogs is compulsory, coverage rarely exceeds 50%. In addition, the long-term maintenance of programmes often remains a problem.

A factor hindering the extermination of rabies in some parts of Asia is the Buddhist prohibition of the killing of stray dogs. The immunization of stray dogs might become a feasible alternative if research into oral vaccines is successful.[29]

Where attempts to eradicate rabies are unsuccessful, supplies of human and animal vaccines are often insufficient. Imports of safe modern vaccines often fail to meet demand, and consequently many developing countries manufacture their own vaccines for post-exposure prophylaxis. Using techniques little advanced beyond Pasteur's original method, neurological complications have been estimated between one in

1200 and one in 120 (see Appendix I). Added to the many painful doses required, post-exposure vaccination is often avoided by those potentially exposed to rabies from a bite.[30] While from the European perspective we may consider rabies a diminishing problem and of little threat to humans, it remains a serious source of concern for public health in large areas of the globe with few signs for optimism.

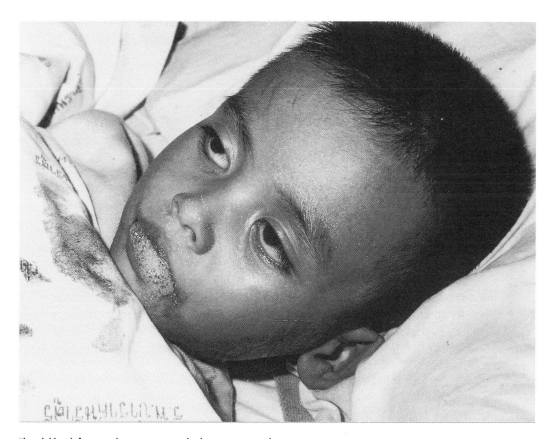

Thai child with furious rabies, sweating and salivating excessively

Rabies-free countries using quarantine

Since May 1993, the *International Animal Health Code* of the Office International des Epizooties (OIE) has defined rabies-free countries as follows.

- The disease is compulsorily notifiable.

- An effective system of disease surveillance is in operation.

- All regulatory measures for the prevention and control of rabies have been implemented including effective importation procedures.

- No case of indigenously acquired rabies infection has been confirmed in man or any animal during the past two years; however, were European Bat Lyssavirus (EBL1 or EBL2) to be identified, this would not affect the country's rabies-free status.

- No imported case in a carnivore has been confirmed outside a quarantine station for the past six months.

The criteria are in agreement with those of WHO and by and large have been adopted or adapted by organizations in the various regions of the world responsible for public or animal health.

Countries reporting no rabies

While the criteria for defining rabies-free status has been generally agreed, the question of which countries meet these criteria has not. Some countries continue to report no rabies, but in the absence of the checks and safeguards set out by the OIE, such as an effective system of surveillance, their 'rabies-free status' will remain in doubt. Without an internationally agreed list of 'rabies-free' countries, it remains the right of importing countries to assess the risk of rabies posed by other countries.

Where there is confidence in rabies surveillance systems, the world may be separated into three groups: countries which have never experienced rabies, countries where rabies has been recorded but the disease has been eradicated and countries where rabies continues to be endemic. Countries in the first group include Australia (although an outbreak of disease considered likely to have been rabies occurred in Tasmania in 1866–7), New Guinea, New Zealand, the State of Hawaii and Antarctica. Examples from the second group include Sweden, where the last documented case was a dog originating from Russia in 1886, Norway (except the islands of Svalbard/Spitzbergen) where the last reported case of rabies was a human case in 1815, Japan and the UK, where the last indigenously acquired human case was in Wales in 1902 and the last animal case was a dog which developed rabies after release from quarantine in 1970.

Hawaii

The policy of the US State of Hawaii, as expressed by the present administration is to be receptive to any alternative to quarantine, if the alternative programme can meet the following criteria:

- offer no less assurance in protecting Hawaii's residents from rabies than quarantine

- incur no additional cost to the residents of Hawaii

- have scientific corroboration.

The decision to change must be based on objective scrutiny of scientific data as well as attention to regulatory concerns. Although the scientific arguments have become more convincing in recent years, such arguments have often not addressed the regulatory concerns. If the requirements of the state policy can be met, the Hawaiian government would take steps to modify its rabies quarantine programme. The aim of this policy is to prevent the introduction of rabies into Hawaii.[31]

At present there is no intention of changing the current 120-day rabies quarantine requirement until the state of Hawaii decides to make changes. Hawaii's situation differs from the UK in that the majority of imported dogs and cats would come from rabies endemic areas such as the USA, whereas in the UK the majority of dog and cat imports would come from EU countries where fox-mediated rabies is either absent or is receding.

Australia

For many years cats and dogs could only be imported from rabies-free countries. Such animals could only be imported by approved routes and had to travel (as they still must) in nose- and paw-proof boxes. Such animals must not have been in a rabies affected country within the previous nine months before release from quarantine in Australia. This was to allow the longest known incubation period to have passed since possible exposure. This led to long quarantine periods and vaccination status played no part in this policy.[32]

In 1993 a national consultation was carried out on a new quarantine policy based on modern diagnostic and vaccine technology. This led to a change in policy. Pet animals are now accepted direct from approved countries (see Table 3) on the basis of control measures and other features

Table 3 Australia's quarantine requirements

Approved rabies-free countries – no quarantine		Approved rabies-free countries – 60 days quarantine	
New Zealand		American Samoa	Niue
Cocos (Keeling) Islands		British Virgin Islands	Papua New Guinea
Norfolk Island		Christmas Island	Solomon Islands
		Cook Islands	Kingdom of Tonga
Approved rabies-free countries – 30 days quarantine		French Polynesia	Tuvalu
Brunei	New Caledonia	Kiribati	Vanuatu
Cyprus	Norway	Nauru	Wallis and Futuna
Fiji	Peninsular Malaysia[a]	Netherlands Antilles	Western Samoa
Finland	Portugal		
Greece	Sabah	**Approved countries and territories recognized by the**	
Hawaii	Sarawak	**Australian Government as countries in which urban**	
Hong Kong	Seychelles	**rabies is absent or well controlled – 120 days quarantine**	
Republic of Ireland	Singapore	Austria	Italy
Japan	Sweden	Belgium	Luxembourg
Malta	Taiwan	Canada	Netherlands
Mauritius	United Kingdom	Denmark	Spain
		France	Switzerland
		Germany	USA
		Greenland	

[a] (excluding designated rabies control area in States of Perlis, Kedah, Perak and Kelantan)

of the disease in those countries. Import of certain particularly aggressive dog breeds (dogo Argentino, fila Brasiliero, Japanese tosa and pit bull terrier or American pit bull) is prohibited. On arrival the animal is transported directly to the quarantine station by quarantine station staff.

Animals imported from approved rabies-free countries and Territories other than New Zealand, Norfolk Island and the Cocos (Keeling) Islands are required to undergo a minimum of 30 or 60 days quarantine at an official animal quarantine station upon arrival, depending on the country of origin. Cats and dogs from approved rabies-free countries do not require pre-export vaccination against rabies.

Animals imported from other approved countries will be required to undergo a minimum of 120 days quarantine at an official animal quarantine station upon arrival. Cats and dogs must have been vaccinated against rabies at least six months and within 12 months prior to export and to have 0.5 IU/ml antibody in their serum. During the quarantine period each animal will be tested for antibody against rabies. Animals with insufficient antibody may be re-exported or destroyed or be required to serve a longer period in quarantine. These changes differ from those envisaged for EU countries in that quarantine still plays a role, although for a much reduced period.

Animals from non-approved countries are not eligible for import directly into Australia but must first spend at least six months in an approved country.

New Zealand

New Zealand has never had a recorded case of rabies. Dogs and cats have been permitted direct entry only from approved rabies-free countries or states such as Australia, Sweden, Norway, UK and Hawaii. Dogs and cats from countries where rabies occurs must stay at least six months in one of these approved rabies-free countries. On entry to New Zealand there are no further restrictions. However, a dog coming from the USA, for example, has two options: it can be imported from Hawaii, where it has been quarantined for four months, followed by a subsequent two month period of residency in the country, or it can come via the UK (six months quarantine) followed by a minimum of two months residency. Similar conditions are required for importation of dogs from canine rabies endemic countries of the world. The policy is to change. The recommendations of the Office International des Epizooties (OIE),

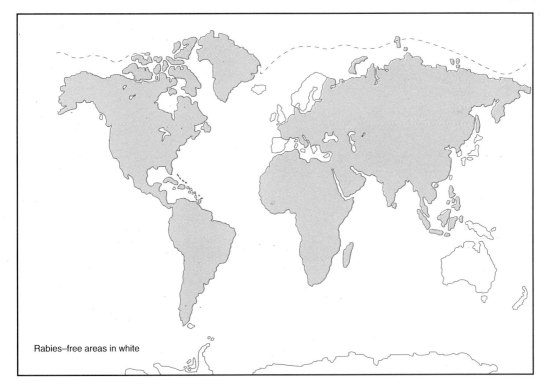

Rabies–free areas in white

Rabies around the world

dated January 1994, have been adopted in principle and a 30 day
quarantine period will be enforced for dogs and cats on arrival in New
Zealand. No quarantine facilities are presently available but dogs and
cats can be quarantined in Australia or Hawaii.[33]

Until recently, the UK played a central and crucial role in the world's
quarantine systems. There is no doubt that attention to the quarantine
procedures of the above three countries has been focused by the pressure
put upon the UK by other EU countries to allow quarantine to be
replaced by vaccination/antibody testing. Hawaii has not yet changed its
policy but Australia and New Zealand have reduced the period of
quarantine, but not abandoned it altogether.

Table 4 lists patterns of rabies around the world.

Table 4 Patterns of rabies around the world

Feature	Europe	Asia	Africa	North America	South and Central America	Arctic rabies[34]
Animals affected: primary vectors	75% of reported rabies cases: red fox (*Vulpes vulpes*) (serotype 1) Turkey: predominantly dog-mediated rabies dog and fox rabies in some areas of Eastern Europe insectivorous bats (European Bat Lyssaviruses genotypes 5 and 6). Bat rabies first diagnosed 1954; apparently rarer than terrestrial rabies but confirmed in more than 400 European bats of at least 8 species	domestic dog (*Canis familiaris*), fox, Arctic fox (*Alopex lagopus*): northern part of former Soviet Union wolf (*Lupus lupus*): some regions of Iran, Afghanistan, Iraq and former Soviet Union	domestic dog thought to represent >75% all animal rabies cases[28] South Africa: black-backed jackals (*Canis mesomelas*), yellow mongoose (*Cynictis penicillata*), bat-eared fox (*Otocyon megalotis*) and dogs in some areas Zambia and Zimbabwe: independent cycle among jackals	91% animal rabies cases in USA among wild animals (1991) Arctic rabies also vectors vary by region: include grey fox (*Urocyon cineroargenteus*); red fox, spotted skunk (*Mephitis mephitis*) and raccoon (*Procyonlotor*) rabies found in 37 species of bat, but no evidence of their starting terrestrial epizootics	vampire bat (*Desmodus rotundus* is most common) dog rabies	arctic rabies (serotype 1 Lyssavirus) is a disease of both wild and domestic animals species: arctic fox (*Alopex lagopus*), red fox, raccoon dog (*Nyctereutes procyonoides*), domestic dog, and possibly wolf and coyote (*Canis latrans*)

Table 4 continued

Feature	Europe	Asia	Africa	North America	South and Central America	Arctic rabies[34]
Animals affected: 'spillover'	domestic animals: dogs, cats, cattle, sheep, goats wild animals: badger (*Meles meles*), raccoon dog (in some countries), deer (*Odocoileus virginianus*), and other mammals	monkeys domestic animals	jackal and hyena important in some parts of Africa domestic animals west Africa: wide 'spillover' infection among wild species	1991: 9% rabies cases in domestic species	foxes, skunks and coyotes among others cattle infected by vampire bats cause huge economic losses (reported 514 000 cattle deaths per annum but true figures much higher)[35]	other animals may be infected, such as prey animals of carnivores listed above
Human cases	terrestrial rabies 1977–1992: 7 indigenously acquired cases in western Europe 115 cases reported in eastern Europe, Turkey and the European part of the former Soviet Union Bat rabies: one case recorded in Finland (1985) and two in Russia[36]	comprehensive/reliable figures unavailable 25 000 deaths per year reported in India (probably underestimate)[13] high incidence human rabies also reported in Bangladesh, Nepal and the many islands of the Philippines	North Africa: deaths estimated 0.4 per 100 000 inhabitants English speaking countries of west Africa: 5–12 deaths per million inhabitants (probably a great underestimate)	US: 10 indigenous cases in last 15 years. Most due to bat rabies virus strains	vast majority of human cases caused by dogs	very few human rabies cases from Arctic rabies Canada: Greenland: 1 since 1960 Alaska: 0 since 1943[37]

Table 4 continued

Feature	Europe	Asia	Africa	North America	South and Central America	Arctic rabies[34]
Prophylaxis for humans	widely available	where rabies vaccine is available, annual number of people receiving post-exposure prophylaxis estimated 800–1000 per million inhabitants per year where dogs are principle vectors[38] three million people treated with post-exposure prophylaxis in India per year[14] Semple vaccine widely used	supplies of human vaccine (often imported) usually fail to meet demand	US: annual rabies prophylaxis 80–90 000 doses Canada: high rate of post-exposure prophylaxis; last human death before 1970	human vaccination rate is very high	low levels of human rabies may be due to occurrence of disease in winter when people are protected by heavy clothing or immunity resulting from hunting methods used in Alaska (see 'further information' at table base)[37]

Table 4 continued

Feature	Europe	Asia	Africa	North America	South and Central America	Arctic rabies[34]
Control measures	large-scale oral vaccination programme of foxes in EU and adjacent countries different policies including vaccination and/or quarantine of imported animals	only countries with considerable resources have succeeded in controlling canine rabies vaccination levels required for dogs are rarely achieved in Asia	control programmes in Algeria, Morocco, Tunisia and Egypt difficulties in maintaining dog vaccination programmes in the long-term	US: vaccination primarily focused on domestic animals; 20–30 million doses given to domestic animals per annum attempts also to vaccinate raccoons Canada: pet and raccoon (wild) vaccination also, plus public health campaign	hundreds of thousands of doses of rabies vaccines sold per annum for rabies vaccination of cattle[39] some success in population reduction of vampire bats. Anti-coagulant drugs, injected into cattle which kill vampire bats but do no harm to the cattle (their food source)	field trials of oral vaccines have proved promising

Table 4 continued

Feature	Europe	Asia	Africa	North America	South and Central America	Arctic rabies[34]
Outlook	advance of epizootic has recently stopped, but causes remain unclear programme of oral vaccination has reduced terrestrial rabies cases but eradication not yet achieved by this method in any country	canine rabies problem is not generally improving and will either remain stable or spread in future years[28]	rabies surveillance hampered by scarcity of diagnostic laboratories increase in animal rabies cases in 1990s in Angola, Algeria, Botswana and Uganda	animal rabies cases rose 24% from 1992, mainly due to increase in raccoon rabies eliminating epizootic from north American wildlife remains formidable task [40]		eradication of Arctic rabies by oral vaccination of wildlife (fox and raccoon dog) is considered feasible, economic and safe[34]
Rabies-infected countries	all of Europe except those listed below	all Asia except for those listed below	In 1993: all Africa except for those listed below	all of North America	all of South and Central America except for those below	Canada, some parts of USA, Greenland, Svalbard Islands of Norway, Poland and former Soviet Union
Countries reporting no rabies	in first half of 1994: Denmark, Netherlands and Luxembourg	no data available for China or most of India	Libya		no information for: Argentina, Costa Rica, Nicaragua	not applicable

Table 4 continued

Feature	Europe	Asia	Africa	North America	South and Central America	Arctic rabies[34]
Rabies-free countries (no indigenous case for at least two years)	UK, Finland, Greece, Ireland, mainland of Norway, Portugal, mainland and islands of Spain, Sweden and Iceland	Bahrain, Japan, Maldives, Qatar, Tonga, Taiwan, Singapore and some Pacific Islands e.g. Bali, Solomon Islands, Papua New Guinea	Mauritius, Seychelles		Antigua/Barbados, Bahamas, Saint Lucia	not applicable
Further information		rabies is common in Asia, but accurate information is rare; 96% of human cases and 93% of animal cases are diagnosed on clinical grounds only which are less reliable			some Caribbean islands e.g. Cuba, Grenada, Dominican Republic, Puerto Rico suffer from mongoose rabies[41]

vampire bat rabies: Trinidad and Tobago | Finland, now rabies-free suffered an outbreak of Arctic rabies in 1988, but successfully eradicated it through oral immunization of raccoon dogs and foxes

case reported of Arctic fox trapper in Alaska developing antibodies to rabies above 0.5 IU without vaccination or infection[37] |

Australasia and Antarctica are rabies-free.

Chapter 4

Recent developments

The European Union

One of the aims of the European Union, as enshrined in the Treaty Establishing the European Community (formerly known as the Treaty of Rome) is to promote the free movement of goods, services, people and capital between the member nations. In the eyes of the European Commission (the secretariat of the European Council) import controls, such as the use of quarantine, and the diseases that make such controls necessary, stand in the path of this aim. The Commission's policy is two-fold: to provide funding for the eradication of rabies from Europe and its immediate borders to the east and to harmonize the rules which govern the movement of goods and people between EU nations. This applies to other veterinary diseases as well as rabies. Were rabies to be eradicated from Europe it is anticipated that pressure would be placed upon Britain to withdraw quarantine restrictions for animals from the EU, though it would remain for animals entering Britain from outside the EU.

However, there is some evidence that the Commission's emphasis on the free movement of animals has already proved detrimental to the health of animals in Britain. Until 1 January 1993 when trade barriers were lifted throughout the European Union, the responsibility for health certification and identification lay with the importing country. However, since this date, the responsibility now resides with the exporter and there are fears that less care and vigilance is exercised since an exported animal presents no risk to the exporting nation.

This freedom of movement between member states does not just open Britain's door to EU nations, but even wider: livestock imported into a member state from outside the Union may then be transported to Britain without further checks. One of the greatest rabies threats to western Europe is thought to be the movement of livestock from former Eastern Bloc countries into the EU.

In 1993 warble fly, an infestation of cattle, which had been eradicated from the UK in 1991, was imported in cattle from France. It is thought that the error in importing the infested cattle may have been due to confusion in terminology used by the French and UK veterinary professions in the animals' certification. Before the removal of the EU's internal borders, all livestock entered quarantine, and many were treated there for warbles.[42]

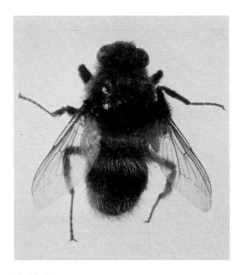

Warble fly

European Union law requires that, other things being equal, all member states must permit and facilitate the free movement of people, goods and services.[43] However, it is widely and mistakenly believed that any border checks are contrary to EU law; restrictions on the free movement of, for example, pets and other animals *are* permissible if they are necessary for the protection of the public health.[44] Thus, at present, Britain has the right to check European Union citizens for pets and commercially traded dogs and cats when entering the UK and it would contravene European law to bring animals subject to quarantine or rabies vaccination (commercially traded cats and dogs) into the UK without complying with those regulations. Following a ruling of the European Court of Justice, any restrictions imposed by a member state on movement within the EU must satisfy the criteria of being both non-discriminatory and proportional.[45] Proportionality means, in effect, that no member state may use regulations disproportionate to the risk involved. Restrictions imposed must be the minimum necessary to deal adequately with the risk posed to health. A set of regulations would be discriminatory if it applied in different ways to non-British owned pets from the way it applied to British owned animals.

If a member state believes it has public health grounds to impose procedures which disrupt free movement under article 36 of the Treaty of Rome, as amended by the Single European Act, it must demonstrate to the Commission that its actions are justified.[46] This evidence must then be reviewed by the European Commission, and either endorsed and applied throughout the EU, or rejected and the restrictions dismantled. As long as they are deemed to conform to these conditions, border checks for smuggled animals or those not fulfilling the requirements of the Rabies (Importation of Dogs, Cats and Other Mammals) Order 1974 (as amended), should continue to be legal within EU law.

The provision for the protection of public health has since been strengthened through Article 129 of the Maastricht Treaty which sets out a new remit in public health for the EU. Thus in drafting legislation, the European Commission must not only consider the implications for trade, but must work towards improvements in public health.

Development of oral vaccines for foxes and other animals

The strain of rabies virus prevalent in most of Europe is carried primarily by the red fox *(Vulpes vulpes)*, which forms a wildlife reservoir for the virus, which can spread into domestic animal populations. As domestic animals and pets are relatively easy to control, there would be great benefits gained from the eradication of rabies in wildlife. However, attempts to remove this wildlife reservoir by killing the foxes themselves, through poisoning, trapping and gassing have had limited success; instead, the immunization of foxes against rabies may provide the answer.

The possibility of controlling rabies in wildlife by immunization has been vigorously investigated for more than 30 years. In the 1970s a breakthrough was made in rabies vaccination techniques with the development of an oral vaccine containing live attenuated rabies virus. The aim of oral vaccination of foxes was to make sufficient numbers immune to interrupt the chain of transmission, leading eventually to the eradication of the wildlife virus's reservoir from Europe. This prospect now appears to be much closer.

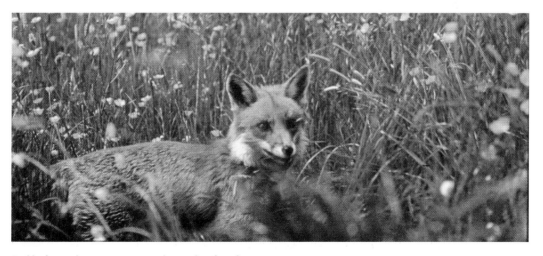

Healthy fox: oral vaccination may eradicate rabies from foxes in Europe

There are currently four types of oral vaccines in use: the three live attenuated rabies viruses, SAD Bern, SAD B19 and SAG2, and a genetically engineered recombinant vaccine in which the glycoprotein gene of the rabies virus is inserted in the genome of the vaccinia virus. These oral vaccines probably infect the animals through contact with the mucous membranes of the mouth and throat.[47]

The vaccination programme

In 1978 the first field study of the attenuated rabies virus oral vaccine was carried out in Switzerland (SAD Bern virus was used). Capsules of the vaccine were placed inside bait of severed chicken heads, 52 000 of which were distributed in various vaccination zones over a period of four years.[48] This study demonstrated that the chain of infection among fox populations could be interrupted. Immunity was induced in 60% of foxes and rabies was eradicated from 80% of Switzerland.[49] Several further trials took place in the then Federal Republic of Germany in 1983.[47] Machine-manufactured sausage-like baits distributed by helicopter accelerated the progress of vaccination campaigns in Italy, Austria, Belgium, France and Luxembourg.

Field trials with the vaccinia recombinant vaccine began in Belgium in 1989 and were extended to France in 1990.[50] No complications have been reported.[50] Following these pilot studies, the European Commission has co-ordinated and largely funded a massive programme of fox vaccination, sharing the cost with national authorities. Started in autumn 1989, the programme aims to eliminate rabies from all European (including non-EU) countries. However, no attempts have been made to control bat rabies. Rabid bats are not responsible for establishing epizootics among terrestrial animals in Europe and therefore pose no threat to other wildlife or pets. It is unlikely that a European country's rabies-free status, as defined by the WHO, would be affected by the presence of rabies in its bats.

How successful has the programme been so far? Oral vaccination in Europe has undoubtedly reduced the incidence of wildlife rabies. Between 1989 and 1992 the number of rabid wild animals reported fell by more than 50%.[51] This trend is seen most dramatically in France.[52] Following an outbreak Finland eradicated the disease by a combination of vaccination and destruction of wildlife. Switzerland eradicated rabies, but subsequently reported re-infection from adjacent countries.

Co-operation with adjoining countries is essential to combat the problems of reintroduction of the virus. Vaccination campaigns have lacked co-ordination across and even within countries, as in the case of some German states, and this has been blamed for the mixed success of previous campaigns. The European Commission states that it will no longer fund the vaccination campaigns of countries which do not co-ordinate their efforts with neighbouring nations.[53] To prevent re-infection, in 1993 the European Commission also paid half of the costs of campaigns in the border regions of the Czech Republic and Austria. In 1994 there were plans to extend the rabies-free belt to Poland, Slovakia, Hungary and Slovenia. The most recent campaign (started in April 1994)

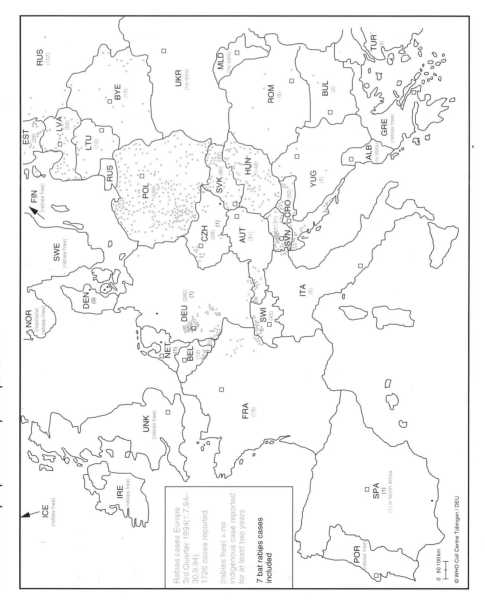

Rabies cases in Europe reported for 1 July–30 September 1994

Rabies cases Europe
3rd Quarter 1994 (1.7.94–30.9.94)
1726 cases reported

(rabies free) = no
indigenous case reported
for at least two years

7 bat rabies cases
included

0 50 100km

© WHO Coll Centre Tübingen / DEU

aims to rid the EU of terrestrial rabies within four years, pushing back the frontiers of rabies-affected areas to eastern Europe.

However, the programme has recently encountered further setbacks. In 1994 Germany, the EU state with the highest rabies incidence, did not maintain its rapid rate of reduction of fox rabies. While France continues to report few cases, Table 5 shows the scale of what remains to be achieved in Germany.

Table 5 Animal rabies in Germany and France 1989–1994[a]

	Domesticated animals				Wild animals					Total
	dog	cat	other[b]	total	fox	deer	badger	other[c]	total	
Germany										
1989	163	329	754	1246	4855	316	128	278	5577	6823
1990	192	267	523	1082	3937	242	94	216	4489	5571
1991	153	189	282	624	2665	130	48	132	2975	3599
1992	59	77	138	274	1011	56	24	60	1151	1425
1993	6	25	110	141	636	28	16	24	704	845
1994[d] incomplete	(5)	(17)	(101)	(123)	(726)	(28)	(24)	(15)	(793)	(916)
France										
1989	53	117	554	724	3341	28	35	86	3490	4214
1990	50	82	331	463	2406	19	37	59	2521	2984
1991	38	83	269	390	1663	24	23	45	1755	2165
1992	30	49	138	217	1000	16	16	35	1067	1284
1993	4	11	26	41	198	1	6	15	220	261
1994[d] incomplete	(1)	(1)	(13)	(15)	(67)	(0)	(1)	(5)	(73)	(88)

[a] Figures derived from WHO Rabies Bulletin Europe 1989–September 1994
[b] Includes cattle, sheep, goats, horses
[c] Includes wild cat, raccoon, raccoon dog, wild boar, squirrel, bat
[d] January 1 1994–September 30 1994

It has been argued that if the European fox vaccination programme is successful, and rabies is eradicated, quarantine could be replaced by a system of animal vaccination for animals travelling between EU countries, including Britain. Yet there remain obstacles to be overcome.[54]

Releasing vaccines containing live virus into the environment has proved controversial as the viruses could theoretically revert to their virulent forms. In the case of the live attenuated rabies virus, a wild mammal might become rabid. Although there is no possibility that the vaccinia recombinant vaccine could cause rabies infection, there have been reservations about the use of the vaccinia virus as a vector. This was partly because of the history of side effects associated with smallpox vaccination and partly because its pathogenesis (ability to produce disease), and its spread and behaviour when introduced into nature are uncertain. However, the deletion of the thymidine kinase gene in the recombinant virus dramatically reduces the pathogenicity of the parent vaccinia virus. Many animals may become infected with a variety of pox viruses naturally and these viruses could theoretically recombine with the vaccinia recombinant to produce a virus of unknown pathogenicity and virulence. The probability of such an occurrence has been estimated to be one in several million animals vaccinated. Other pox viruses are also being developed as recombinant vaccines with rabies glycoprotein.

Were the current programmes of oral vaccination of foxes to succeed in eradicating rabies from Europe, the question remains whether another animal could take the fox's place in the spread of rabies.

The bat

There is no evidence that infected bats have initiated epizootics of rabies in terrestrial mammals. European bat Lyssaviruses (EBL) are clearly distinguishable from serotype 1 rabies viruses, and no EBL has been reported in a terrestrial animal to date, although relatively few specimens have been examined.[55]

The raccoon dog

One possible candidate for replacing the red fox as vector and reservoir of the rabies virus is the raccoon dog (*Nyctereutes procyonoides*), which was introduced from eastern Asia into Russia and has spread into Lithuania, Sweden, Poland and Germany. In parts of Russia and Poland it is an increasingly important host of the rabies virus, and in these countries the species may already be a reservoir of the disease.

However, if raccoon dogs were to replace the red fox as the primary vector and reservoir of rabies, oral vaccination would probably eradicate the disease once more. Finland's experience proves the efficacy of oral vaccination in this species and field trials in Lithuania were successful.[56]

The wolf

Wolves are highly susceptible to rabies and attempts to re-establish the species in western Europe may have significant implications for the disease's spread. In Russia the wolf population is increasing and wolf rabies presents a significant problem. Primitive methods of control through extermination are being employed, but oral vaccination, as used for foxes, has not been tried.

If the population density of an animal is below a certain level, the chances of rabies spreading are low. However, due to the work of conservationists, wolf numbers are increasing in Sweden, Norway, the former Soviet Union, Poland, Germany, the Czech Republic, Slovakia, Hungary, Romania and Italy. Attempts are also being made to link geographically isolated wolf populations, which could further aid the transmission of the virus across Europe.

Whether the vaccines could be used effectively among all the potential vectors and reservoirs of rabies is unclear. It is probable that some adjustment to the vaccine strength would be required and the baits made attractive to other species.

The Channel Tunnel

As an island, Britain's natural defences have helped her to remain free of rabies. Many fear that the creation of a permanent link with mainland Europe will threaten that status, mere mention of the tunnel prompting visions of rabid animals making their way under the Channel into Britain.

The Channel Tunnel consists of three separate tunnels: one in each direction for trains and a third service tunnel. A multi-layered defence system has been built for Eurotunnel, who in 1987 gave an undertaking to comply with the Government's requirements of 1985 to keep rabies out of Britain. But many people are asking whether these precautions are sufficient. Questions have been raised as to whether animals could inhabit the tunnels or stow away in or underneath the trains; whether rabid foxes could inhabit the area of the tunnel's mouth in France, or bats fly through or colonize the tunnels.

With the emotional response generated by such discussion, the issues need to be placed in perspective. First, the area of France around the tunnel, Coquelle near Calais, has no endemic rabies. Furthermore, rabies is declining in France due to the programmes of oral vaccination of foxes and cases of rabies in northern France are very rare: in 1991 two rabid foxes were isolated about one hundred miles south of the tunnel's mouth along the River Somme (Départment de Pas-de-Calais) and more recently in 1994 one rabid fox was found near Paris (over 100 miles from the tunnel), an area free of the disease during the previous two years.[57]

Given these grounds for a rabies threat, there are three possibilities for transmission of the virus via the tunnel to the English animal population: an animal making its way across country towards the tunnel beyond the normal area of rabies incidence; the front of rabies moving towards the French tunnel mouth; or an animal smuggled through the tunnel.

The first case envisages a fox travelling far from its territory and through the tunnel: foxes suffering from furious rabies may travel considerable distances, but foxes usually develop the paralytic furious form of the disease which tends to make them apathetic and inhibits movement outside their original territory.[11,58,59] It is therefore unlikely that the animal would be a fox, and most dogs and cats in rabies-enzootic areas of France are vaccinated against rabies.

The second possibility involves the front of rabies infections moving towards the mouth of the Channel Tunnel. The French veterinary service has formally agreed with the British veterinary service at Tolworth and the Standing Veterinary Committee of the European Commission, to intensify its programme of oral vaccination of wild foxes in the Pas-de-Calais were any such movement detected. To guard against any animal entering the tunnel a multi-layered defence system has been constructed in and around the tunnel, comprising fences, electrical deterrents, poisoned baits and patrols of the entrances.

A three tier system has been installed against the passage of animals through the tunnels. The first defence is a perimeter fence of animal-proof mesh three metres high topped with two feet of razor wire and buried below ground. Poison baits are laid along the base of the fence. The perimeter fence in England surrounds the entire mouth of the tunnel with the exception of three entrances for trains, cars and personnel which are under closed circuit TV 24 hours a day. In France the perimeter fence is ten miles long and of the same animal-proof design.

The second barrier consists of the portal fence of similar design to the perimeter fence but closer to the mouths of the tunnels, extending 200

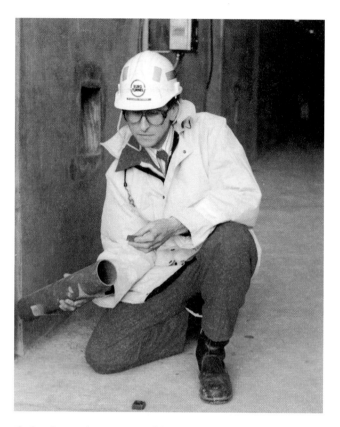

Checking baits at the UK entrance of the Channel Tunnel

yards along the track. While it is not possible to seal the tunnels from animals, the late Mr Anthony Crowley, Veterinary Consultant to Eurotunnel and former MAFF rabies control section head, contended that it would be an extremely determined animal that succeeded in getting round this and the previous fence, the poisoned baits and not be deterred by the bright lights and noise at the tunnel mouths. Furthermore, the portal fencing is duplicated at the mouth of the French side of the tunnels.

The third level of defence consists of electrified grids at the end of the undersea sections of the three tunnels. Similar to cattle grids, and alternatively earthed and electrified, they carry a voltage sufficient to deter rather than kill animals and when tested against rats have been successful. A mock-up of the defences were tested at the Centre National d'Etudes Vétérinaires et Alimentaires (CNEVA) in Nancy, France, against healthy rats, cats, and dogs and both rabid and healthy foxes; in Britain they were tested against healthy rats and in all tests no animal succeeded in breaching the barriers. This electrified grid runs across the floor of the tunnel. In the case of the evacuation of passengers the grid can be switched off to allow them to cross, but a warning device should prevent them being left off for any length of time. Bulkheads connected electrically to the grids are designed to prevent animals passing across pipes and cables. In total there are six barriers for an animal to cross in addition to the 31 miles of tunnel it would need to pass through.

The possibility of small animals such as rodents running along the rails has not been fully solved, but the likelihood of their survival in such a hostile environment is remote. There are poisoned baits throughout the tunnel; any animal stowed beneath the train would be crushed; Eurotunnel's shuttle trains are hermetically sealed allowing no fodder to

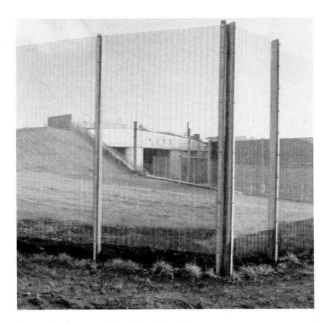

Security fencing around the Channel Tunnel

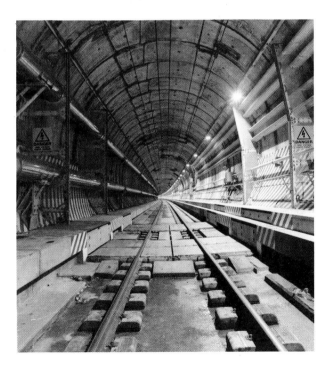

Electrified grids on the floor of the Channel Tunnel

escape which could encourage animals; toilets on the trains are sealed tanks and the tunnels' drains are all meshed to prevent animals entering them. All passenger trains passing through the tunnel will have to conform to these requirements. Rats, while able to carry the disease, have never been known to cause an outbreak of rabies, so any risk they might present of reintroducing rabies to Britain is purely theoretical. During its construction, only two rats were spotted in the tunnel both of which were destroyed.

According to MAFF, the frequency with which the high speed trains will pass through the tunnel will discourage most animals from attempting to get through and the air turbulence caused by the trains will make it virtually impossible for bats to fly through the tunnel.[24] Eurotunnel has given an undertaking that its inspection systems will keep all animals out of the trains.

The tunnels are inspected daily for colonization by bats which, as a protected species, cannot be killed, but would instead be removed. No bats have been found in the tunnels. The question has been raised whether bats could fly down the service tunnel which does not accommodate trains but this tunnel is safeguarded from animals by double airlocks at

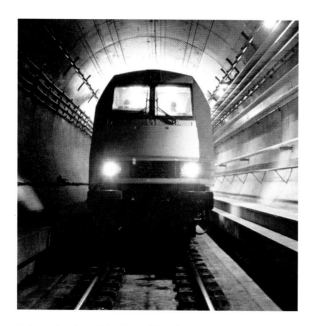

Train passing through the Channel Tunnel

each end. These doors are opened several times a day for the service tunnel vehicles, but each time this occurs, the outer door is opened and then closed behind the vehicle and the inner door is only opened once the chamber has been checked for animals.

If an animal is found inside the tunnels or terminal areas, teams from Kent County Council will be called to catch it. These teams, and the personnel laying and servicing the tunnels' poison baits, will have been vaccinated against rabies.

The defences against rabid animals passing by their own efforts through the Channel Tunnel appear very secure. However, the most likely route for rabies to reach Britain is by smuggling. It is reassuring that Eurotunnel has precautions against smuggling. Eurotunnel's shuttle trains will carry no pets, livestock or animals of any kind; traffic is monitored for smuggled animals and any found will be impounded in animal pens at the terminals.

Concern has been raised over the freedom of lorries to drive directly on to the British motorways without passing the port health inspectors. The responsibility for checking cargo has been transferred from the health inspectors of the port of entry to local authority staff at the lorry's destination. Such local authorities may be inexperienced in carrying out the necessary checks and surveillance, and by the time the lorry has reached its destination the smuggled animal may have escaped into the countryside.

The rabies threat posed by animals passing through the Channel Tunnel without human assistance appears no greater, and possibly smaller, than that of more traditional forms of cross-channel travel. The main danger is likely to arise from smuggling – the intentional circumventing of rabies control measures. While border checks at British ports have become less stringent, the threat from animals smuggled in boats and via the tunnel remains a significant one.

Chapter 5

Smuggling

Animals may be smuggled into Britain from an EU member state, from outside Europe, or, capitalizing on the freer movement possible within the EU, from a third country via an EU member state. Since the introduction of the single market on 1 January 1993, movement into Britain from outside the Union has been subject to the same scrutiny as before, but within EU borders, there have been significant changes. Anecdotal evidence suggests few obstacles face those attempting to avoid quarantine by smuggling animals, particularly by car, from France to Britain.

Responsibility for control

When traffic passes into a British port or airport from a European member state, HM Customs and Excise may no longer carry out routine checks, but only random 'spot checks'. Although they are not directly responsible for preventing the entry of unauthorized rabies susceptible animals such as cats and dogs into Britain, they do have the power to withhold clearance on unlicensed animals for control by other enforcement agencies. In practice this means that if, while customs staff are examining a person or luggage for illegal substances such as narcotics, they discover a stowed animal, they will prevent its further passage and call in the local authority responsible or the Crown Prosecution Service to consider prosecution. However, the opportunities to carry out such checks on those coming from EU member states are now greatly reduced. Anyone who has passed through the 'blue channel' for EU travellers will know how rarely checks are now made.

The enforcement of public health controls, including the import of animals, is the responsibility of local authorities. Illegal landings of rabies susceptible animals fall within the jurisdiction of the local authority in which they occur. Those authorities responsible for ports or airports are represented by the Association of Port Health Authorities (APHA). In a memorandum to the Commons Select Committee on Agriculture, the APHA states:

> Since the completion of the internal market, checks by customs officers and port health officers on traffic arriving from other member states in the European Union have virtually ceased, and we are concerned that there are virtually no checks to prevent the illegal importation of cats and dogs by people arriving from the EU....it is now very easy for travellers in Europe to pick up a stray cat or dog which could be infected with rabies and bring it back to the UK where the animal population is largely unprotected against the disease.[60]

Although reported cases of rabies are relatively rare among pet animals in Europe, the removal of internal frontiers in Europe also raises the risk from countries outside the EU. Once an animal has passed into the EU, free movement between member states and into Britain is considerably easier. A major danger is posed by animals imported from rabies-endemic nations into EU nations which have no quarantine regulations. They may then be smuggled into Britain, with relative ease, through Customs' 'blue channel' as EU traffic.

In addition to the greatly reduced surveillance of traffic entering Britain from EU nations, a further source of concern is the recent announcement of job cuts in HM Customs and Excise. Staff numbers will fall from just over 25 000 to 21 000 by 1999. This reduction includes 600 anti-smuggling officers, who staff entry points at airports and ports.

Such a state of affairs is extremely worrying from the point of view of retaining Britain's rabies-free status as smuggling is likely to be made easier. The single market will aid illegal movements both from EU member states and from countries outside the EU. The reduction in anti-smuggling officers from HM Customs and Excise will increase further the risk of rabies entering Britain from the rest of the world. If regulations are to be effective, whether by vaccination and certification or quarantine, smuggling must be prevented.

Motives for smuggling

The debate on smuggling is bedevilled by the lack of hard evidence, either of its incidence or the motives behind the act. Those accused of smuggling may defend themselves by pleas of ignorance of the regulations, rather than divulge the truth. We know that between 1985 and 1993, HM Customs and Excise detected 492 cases of illegal entry of dogs and 273 involving cats (see Table 6). But obviously, an unknown number are successfully brought in. Estimates put it at between one hundredth and one tenth of the true figure. Conflicting theories have been proposed regarding possible motives for smuggling and on how a change in policy might influence smuggling behaviour.

Table 6 Imports of rabies susceptible animals into Britain, 1985–93

| Year | Illegal Landings | | | Prosecutions | | |
	dogs	cats	other mammals	dogs and cats	other mammals	results (max. fine, £)
1985	44	36	109 (in 21 batches)	72	5	1500
1986	50	27	34 (in 18 batches)	62	13	1200
1987	26	25	92 (in 17 batches)	34	8	1000
1988	93	16	75 (in 16 batches)	54	2	1500
1989	38	28	93 (in 13 batches)	25	4	1600
1990	59	40	92 (in 12 batches)	43	2	1000
1991	72	39	23 (in 16 batches)	57	7	2000
1992	60	33	46 (in 11 batches)	40	5	1250
1993	50	39	56 (in 13 batches)	22	2	1200

It has been argued that the expense and separation from a beloved pet caused by quarantine are significant motivations for animal smuggling and that replacement with a cheaper system of vaccination and identification, with no period of isolation, would reduce the incentive to smuggle.[61] However, it could equally be argued that such a change in policy could be interpreted as the relaxation or even abolition of Britain's rabies defences. Indeed, such a perception has already been indicated by the press. The Balai Directive on the replacement of quarantine with vaccination and identification for traded animals was followed by headlines such as 'Quarantine rules change as rabies defences weaken' and the recommendations for vaccination and identification of the Commons Select Committee on Agriculture were reported as 'Britain should drop control on rabies, says MPs'.[61-63] If such a perception is widely held, the threat posed by rabies may be underestimated and animal smuggling may actually increase.

As we have already seen, smuggling between EU nations is relatively straightforward. It can be mistakenly assumed that compared with quarantine, vaccination is a simple procedure and for this reason less likely to encourage illegal avoidance. But it is unlikely that an individual who is prepared to ignore all warnings of the dangers of smuggling a pet into Britain and risk introducing rabies will be willing to follow the complex procedures involved in, for example, the system recommended by the Commons Select Committee on Agriculture. A risk assessment of Sweden's then proposed vaccination system, carried out by the Swedish Board of Agriculture, concluded 'It is by no means self-evident that smuggling will be reduced if the rules are altered'.[64] The prevention of smuggling must be made the primary priority of any anti-rabies policy.

Although the true scale of smuggling of animals into Britain is unknown, it probably poses the greatest threat to our rabies-free status. Greater measures should be taken to deter and prevent smuggling. The fines listed in Table 6 for 1993 amount to less than the fees for one dog in quarantine. Unless the penalties are substantially increased, smuggling will remain a risk worth taking.

While rabies remains a risk to Britain, border checks against smuggling remain in accordance with the provisions of the Treaty Establishing the European Community for the protection of public health. However, if there are to be fewer customs officers, alternative means of detecting smuggled animals must be found. Heat-sensitive cameras, for instance, could be used to detect animals stowed in vehicles or luggage on ferries or trains. With the money and effort invested in keeping rabies out of Britain, it would be lamentable if it took an outbreak of rabies for the risk of smuggling to be taken seriously.

Chapter 6

Dealing with an outbreak of rabies in Britain

Understanding the threat of rabies

When considering the threat which rabies poses to British wildlife, there are a number of questions to be answered.

- How quickly would it spread?

- Could we eradicate a limited outbreak of the disease?

- Although we succeeded in eradicating rabies early this century, would this be possible once the disease was established?

To answer these questions we need to understand how Britain's habitat and animal populations have changed since the nineteenth century. We will also examine how animals behave and interact while healthy and when rabid.

An important feature of the disease in either its dumb or furious form, is that wild animals that are normally wary will lose their fear when infected and approach other animals and humans much more closely, and they may even enter farm buildings and houses. Other behaviour patterns may also be affected; for instance animals which are normally nocturnal may start to wander around in daylight.

Transmission of the rabies virus by saliva, the most important route in the spread of the disease, occurs most commonly among animals by biting during fights. However, transmission can also occur during social grooming or from an aerosol in enclosed spaces, as virus particles can be excreted in the water droplets in exhaled breath. Thus the social canids, those species in the family Canidae (foxes, jackals, wild dogs, wolves, etc.) that live in social groups, are particularly good hosts for the disease: they actively defend a territory, within the group they mutually groom, and they often share an underground burrow system. The speed with which the disease will spread is in part therefore determined by the social behaviour of the infected individuals. The likelihood of the disease spreading to man is determined by the chance of making contact with the

main host species in a particular area. Domestic animals, especially dogs
and cats, provide the links of infection between wildlife and man.

Changes in British and European fox populations

While the cycle of rabies currently endemic in western mainland Europe
is the sylvatic one, in which the red fox acts as the main vector, the
situation was very different during the last century, when the red fox was
not a particularly important vector in Europe. One theory attributes this
to the large numbers of dogs associated with human settlements in the
countryside of continental Europe. It is believed that the dogs initially
restricted the distribution and abundance of foxes, and there is some
evidence to support this idea from studies in British cities, where foxes
avoid those urban areas where stray dogs are most common. However,
as industrialization and urbanization occurred, and people migrated to
the towns and cities, the numbers of dogs in the countryside fell, and the
rural fox population consequently grew.[65]

While the fox was not a significant rabies vector in nineteenth-century
continental Europe, the same was true for Britain at that time, but the
reasons behind this differed. Until the First World War, there were many
gamekeepers in Britain, who reduced the numbers of all predators in the
countryside, including foxes. Thus it is probable that in Britain foxes
were so thinly distributed that rabies did not enter the fox population or,
if it did, fox densities were too low for the disease to persist.

Since the Second World War, in common with the rest of western
Europe, Britain has seen a growth in its fox population. This increase has
been due to a number of factors, including the decline in the number of
gamekeepers, associated changes in the patterns of mortality caused by
man and an increase in food availability, especially the recovery of rabbit
populations from myxomatosis, and the large numbers of pheasants that
are now being reared and released by the shooting industry. Growth in
the fox population has also been due to spread into areas where they
were, until recently, rare or absent, for example in much of Norfolk and
Suffolk, parts of Dyfed and Gwynedd, and much of the coastal area of
Scotland from Aberdeen to Nairn. The most marked change this century
has been the colonization of new habitats, especially upland coniferous
woodlands and urban areas. Foxes began to colonize areas of low-
density owner-occupied housing in British cities from the 1930s.[66]

Rabies will only persist when the vector population occurs above a
threshold density. As foxes live in family groups, densities are normally
expressed as the number of family groups per km^2. In rural areas of the
western European mainland fox densities are now commonly around 0.3

to 0.5 family groups per km², although densities as high as 1.25 groups per km² have been recorded.[67] Even these lower densities are sufficient to enable the sylvatic cycle of the disease to be maintained by the red fox alone throughout western Europe.

Although only 14% of the country's fox population, Britain's urban foxes have densities among the highest recorded anywhere in the world, and considerably higher than those found in rural areas of Britain, or in areas of mainland Europe which are ahead of the rabies front and therefore still unaffected by the disease. Urban foxes are mainly found south of Nottingham, although there are also populations in Edinburgh and Glasgow. In urban areas, densities frequently exceed one group per km², and may be as high as five groups per km².[68] The presence of the potential main reservoir species for the sylvatic form of the disease at such high densities in many urban areas and living in such close proximity to man and his domestic pets is a situation encountered nowhere else in Europe or North America.

Potential sources for re-introducing rabies to Britain

With the exception of the years 1918–22 and the two isolated cases in 1969 (Camberley) and 1970 (Newmarket), the insularity of Britain and its stringent quarantine regulations have kept the country free of rabies since 1902.[2] However, the greater movement of people between countries, a marked increase in the number of marinas and pleasure craft on the south coast of Britain and recent relaxations in border controls within the European Union, mean that the possibility of an animal being smuggled into Britain is probably higher now than at any time since the Second World War.

Smuggled pet animals

By far the most likely entry route for rabies into Britain would be via an infected pet, most probably a dog or cat, that has been illegally imported. Nearly 80% of the people in Britain live in urban areas with a population size greater than 10 000, and over 50% in urban areas with a population of over 100 000.[69] It is most likely, therefore, that any ensuing rabies epizootic would originate in a large town or city, as that is the most likely destination of a smuggled pet. However, the disease could appear in any part of Britain, and so MAFF has designed rabies control strategies for both rural and urban areas.

The threat to the British fox population

Despite these plans, there is as yet no consensus on whether a British fox could be infected by a dog or cat carrying the European fox-adapted strain of the virus. In any one area, rabies tends to be concentrated in one major host species with only occasional spillover into other species. The reasons behind this 'compartmentation' are not fully understood, but it may be due to adaption of the strain of the rabies virus to its host species. The amount of virus secreted in the saliva of the principal vector may differ in its effects on different species. For instance, were a rabid dog in India – where it is the main rabies vector – to bite another dog, it would be highly likely to cause rabies and the dog bitten would then secrete enough virus in its own saliva to infect another dog. However, were the rabid dog to bite a monkey, the monkey might become an 'end-host', developing the disease but producing little virus in its saliva and so be unlikely to infect another animal. This is possibly partly due to inter-species differences in reactions to the virus. However, there may also be structural differences between the strains of the virus found in different species or different geographical regions.[70]

The fox-adapted rabies strain prevalent throughout western Europe is considered to be poorly transmissible within other species and it has never been documented that dogs or cats have spread the fox-adapted rabies virus into new areas. This concept is of significance for UK quarantine because if correct, it means that dogs and cats imported from the EU may be unlikely to transmit rabies virus into UK wildlife. However, dogs and cats can be infected with a fox-adapted rabies virus, although a large amount is needed. Once infected, there is a 20–30% chance of finding virus in the dog's saliva and a 70–80% chance in cats.[71] This virus could be transferred to a British fox and then into the wider fox population.

Could migrating bats introduce rabies into Britain?

One theoretically possible route for rabies to enter Britain from the continent is via an infected bat. In Europe, there have been three human deaths known to have been associated with bat rabies in the last 30 years, two in the former Soviet Union, and one in Finland.[55] Bat rabies in Europe is primarily confined to serotine bats (*Eptesicus serotinus*), although infected animals from six other species have also been found. The disease is mainly found in bats from Holland, the maritime parts of northern Germany, and Denmark. Although the number of rabies-positive bats is generally small, in one year 28 per cent of serotine bats examined in Denmark were found to be infected.[55] Regular migrations of bats between Britain and continental Europe are thought not to occur, although bats may be blown off course by high winds, and some do appear to reach Britain from the continent.[72] Although serotines have not been sighted flying into Britain from continental Europe, they do fly long distances; as movements of up to 145 and 330 km have been recorded on the continent.[73] It is feasible that one could fly to Britain. However, serotines are not widely distributed in Britain. Population densities are low, and recorded roosts are few and generally confined to the south and south-eastern counties of Hampshire, Surrey and Sussex.[73]

Serotines may share roost sites with other species such as pipistrelles (*Pipistrellus pipistrellus*) and brown long-eared bats (*Plecotus auritus*). Both these species, especially the former, are more abundant than serotines in Britain. However, there is no evidence to suggest that these two species are carriers of the rabies virus to any significant extent.[74] As part of a continuous monitoring programme, material from dead bats found in Britain is submitted to the Central Veterinary Laboratory, Weybridge, for rabies examination. All of more than 1700 bats examined from 15 of the 16 species indigenous to Britain have been negative for rabies. Finally, whilst the type of rabies virus carried by bats will infect and kill man and has killed laboratory rodents, there is no evidence that it can be passed from one terrestrial mammal to another in nature. Thus the likelihood of the disease being transferred to Britain by bats is very small, and most unlikely to lead to a wildlife epizootic.

Measures to control the fox population in a rabies outbreak

The contingency plans for rural and urban areas are basically similar. The prime aim of the current government policy is the containment and elimination of the disease. Since rabies will most probably be introduced via a single smuggled pet, the original focus of infection should be limited in extent. Dealing with this limited point-source infection should, in theory at least, be a lot easier than trying to combat the situation in the rest of Europe, where the disease is widespread and endemic, and the rabies front is over 2000 km long. This fundamental difference explains why the control measures planned for Britain are different from those in use elsewhere.

The Rabies (Control) Order 1974 provides wide powers involving local authorities, the police, and practising veterinary surgeons. The control operation would be co-ordinated by MAFF and the powers used would depend on the actual and potential severity of the outbreak (Table 2, p. 23).

DISEASES OF ANIMALS ACT 1950

THE RABIES (CONTROL) ORDER 1974
(Article 5)

NOTICE DECLARING AND DEFINING THE LIMITS OF AN INFECTED PLACE

To.............................\.......

of ....

I, the undersigned, being an inspector of the Ministry of Agriculture, Fisheries and Food (or an inspector of the local authority for the .... of ....) hereby give you as the occupier of the undermentioned premises notice that in accordance with the provisions of the above-mentioned order, the undermentioned premises are hereby declared to be an infected place for the purposes of the said order, *and that the premises, and any person from time to time thereat, accordingly become subject to the Rules specified in this notice which are printed on the back hereof. Any person infringing these Rules is liable to prosecution.*

This notice remains in force in its present form until it is cancelled or varied by a subsequent notice served by an inspector of the Ministry on the occupier of the infected place.

NOTE.—A notice declaring an infected place may be served under Article 5 of the Rabies (Control) Order in respect of any premises at which there is an animal affected with or suspected of being affected with rabies, or at which such an animal has died, or in respect of premises at which an inspector has reasonable grounds for suspecting that rabies has existed within the previous 56 days, or that there is an animal which has been or which may have been exposed to the infection of rabies through contact with an affected or suspected animal.

Description of infected place

'Declaration of infected place'

Dated......................................19....

(Signed) ....

Official address ....

NOTE.—The Inspector is with all practicable speed to send copies of this notice to the Secretary, Ministry of Agriculture, Fisheries and Food, Animal Health Division, Hook Rise South, Tolworth, Surrey, KT6 7NF, to the local authority, to the Divisional Veterinary Officer and to the police officer in charge of the nearest police station in the district in which the infected place is situated.
The Rules set out in Article 7 are to be printed on the back of this notice.

The premises of an animal suspected of having rabies would be declared an infected place

As soon as it was suspected that an animal was infected with rabies, the premises on which it was kept would be declared an infected place. In many cases, the suspect animal and any contacts would be required to be securely confined within the premises. In some cases, animals might be removed for observation to accommodation maintained by the Agriculture Departments.

If the animal was found to be virus-positive further action would depend on the circumstances. The critical factor would be whether the infected animal could have infected others, including wildlife. If this were the case, the next step would be to declare an infected area, the size of which would again depend on the circumstances. This would enable any or all of the following measures to be put into effect:

- restriction of movement of animals into and out of the area

- control and confinement of animals in the area (e.g. muzzling and leashing of dogs and leashing of cats)

- seizure, detention and disposal of animals not under proper control in the area

- compulsory vaccination of animals

- prohibition of gatherings of animals and sporting and recreational activities, including hunting, the racing or coursing of hounds or dogs, point-to-point meetings and the shooting of game or other wildlife

- the destruction of foxes. [24]

Current control measures in the event of a rabies outbreak in Britain's wildlife would concentrate on the destruction of foxes in the infected area while minimizing the hazard to other species of wildlife and to farm and domestic animals. In most kinds of outbreak, the co-operation and assistance of many government, local authority and other interests, including practising veterinary surgeons, would be called upon to put prepared plans into action. Local authorities have a statutory requirement to draw up a contingency plan for an outbreak of rabies in consultation with the health authority. MAFF reports that several successful local authority exercises have tested contingency plans. Supplies of equipment necessary to contain outbreaks have been tested following suspect cases, where an animal has left quarantine and died with possible clinical signs of rabies. Until the all clear is given by testing the animal's brain (at the Central Veterinary Laboratory, Weybridge), a minor exercise is carried out as a precaution. Publicity material is held in readiness for distribution in an infected area. MAFF asserts that 'The country is therefore well-prepared to counter an outbreak effectively.' However, scientists modelling fox population behaviour think that eradicating an outbreak in wildlife might be more difficult than is suggested by the Ministry.

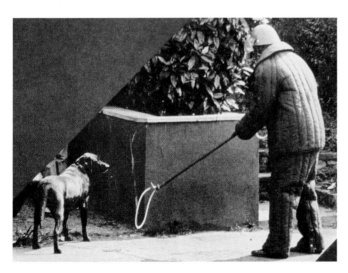

Rabies contingency plans: catching and impounding stray dogs

Oral vaccination as a means of control

The form of control currently practised to combat sylvatic rabies throughout most of western Europe is the oral vaccination of foxes. Although the eradication of rabies from the continent remains a distant prospect, vaccination has been successful in dramatically reducing the number of rabies cases in several countries. This approach is not favoured as a method of control in Britain as a far higher proportion of foxes would require vaccination to break the cycle of infection than in less densely inhabited continental Europe. Field trials carried out in Bristol suggest that uptake of bait was too low to reach the critical level. While mathematical models predict that 75–95% of the British fox population would require vaccination for a rabies outbreak to be controlled, considerably less than this was achieved.[75,76]

To stop the spread of rabies into rabies-free areas and to eradicate the disease from an enzootic area, in field trials in Switzerland between 50% and 80% of all foxes needed immunization. A greater understanding of fox foraging habits may improve the uptake of vaccine baits, but until then, culling remains the control mechanism of choice for MAFF. Furthermore, a culling campaign allows quick and easy risk assessments to be carried out: all foxes seen alive would be potentially rabid (either infected or susceptible to rabies infection) and would therefore need to be killed. With a vaccination programme, there would be no way of knowing from sight alone whether the animal had eaten a vaccine bait, and therefore posed no risk. Time-consuming testing would be required to assess levels of bait uptake and therefore the success of the vaccination campaign, by which time, if it had failed, the disease could have spread a very long way from the original focus and the chance of containment would then be much lower.

Fox population culling

Poison baits will be the main form of control in Britain, and these will be buried just below the ground to minimize eating by species other than the fox. Although the use of poison baits to kill foxes is illegal in Britain under normal circumstances, The Rabies (Control) Order 1974 permits this in a rabies event. An area with a radius of 19 km around the point of infection will be declared a control zone.[77] The boundaries of the control zone will be adjusted to take account of any natural barriers to fox movements, and may be a little smaller in an urban area. In a rabies outbreak, it is important not to disrupt the fox population in such a way as to encourage animals to disperse out of the control zone, as this would accelerate the spread of the disease, hence the prohibition of field sports such as shooting and the hunting of foxes with hounds in the control zone.

Stray dogs and feral cats

While the wildlife control operations are the responsibility of MAFF it is the local authorities that are responsible for the control of domestic animals. In 1993 there were about 6.65 million dogs and 7.18 million

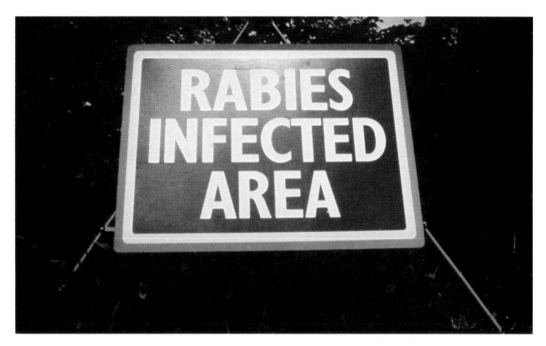

In any outbreak of rabies a control zone would be established swiftly

cats in Britain.[78] Even without rabies, stray dogs are rounded up in British cities because of their nuisance value, and there may be far fewer now than at the end of the last century. However, one estimate suggested that there may be as many as 500 000 stray dogs in Britain, the majority in urban areas.[79] The total feral cat population in Britain is over 800 000, and most are found in rural areas.[80] In urban areas, feral cat colonies are most frequent in Greater London, and the Greater Manchester-Merseyside and West Yorkshire conurbations.[81] As stray dogs and cats are potential vectors of rabies and are more abundant than foxes, they probably have a greater chance of transmitting rabies to humans and/or their pets. It is therefore clearly important to include these in any rabies control operation in both urban and rural areas.

Predicting the pattern of rabies spread in Britain

As we have no experience of the pattern of rabies spread in the high-density fox populations found in British urban areas or, to a lesser extent, parts of rural Britain, it is important that we understand the behaviour of foxes in Britain, and particularly in urban habitats, as this is probably where an outbreak would first appear. Long-term studies over the last 20 years of the ecology of foxes living in Bristol and other British cities have helped us understand, and predict, the behaviour of foxes in different circumstances. Thus methods have been developed to estimate fox densities in any British city simply from the census data and the pattern of land use.[82] Fox density increases with the amount of owner-occupied housing in a town and with the amount of urban fringe land (woodlands, natural parks, farmland, wasteland and other derelict areas occurring within an urban area), but decreases with the amount of council-rented housing, industry, fields and housing occupation density. Obviously, fox numbers are dependent on the availability of food, and the highest numbers occur in residential areas because many householders deliberately put out food for the foxes. In fact foxes living in these areas may obtain half of their energy requirements from householders.[83]

To understand the population biology of urban foxes, capture-mark-recapture techniques have been used to measure fecundity, mortality and the patterns of dispersal of foxes in urban areas.[84,85] A computer simulation model is used to examine the probable pattern of rabies spread and to evaluate the likely success of different control régimes in specific urban areas.[86] This model currently forms the basis of MAFF's rabies control strategy in urban areas, and simulated control operations are undertaken periodically to review the implementation of the contingency plans.

How useful are models for predicting the rate of rabies spread?

One problem with this approach to furthering our understanding of the epizootiology of rabies is that the behaviour of rabies-infected animals may differ greatly from that of healthy ones, and extrapolations based on studies of the behaviour of healthy animals may be inaccurate. However, the limited work that has been done on rabid foxes indicates that although they may start to behave abnormally, they remain approximately faithful to their normal activity areas. Dogs, on the other hand, seem to wander aimlessly under the influence of the virus. Thus, although the number of contacts a fox makes with animals from the same or different groups may be increased by the virus, the animals encountered will be the same as if it were healthy. It is likely then that the contact rate of infected foxes will be similar to that of healthy animals, and so the models are likely to give a realistic assessment of the pattern of rabies spread.

Obtaining accurate predictions of the rate of spread of a disease such as rabies relies on quantified data on the frequency of contacts between individuals of the vector species. The contact rates first used in the model described above were estimates based on those used in previous models which simulated the pattern of rabies spread in Canada. However, recent research has used simultaneous radio-tracking of several urban foxes to try to quantify the actual contacts between animals of the same and different social groups.[87] Intra-group encounters were predominantly non-aggressive and constant in frequency throughout the year. In contrast, inter-group encounters were uncommon and almost always aggressive, although they were much more common in the winter months, when resident males trespassed into neighbouring ranges in search of additional mating opportunities.

Further modelling work enabled contact probabilities at different fox population densities to be derived from these figures. Foxes from neighbouring groups tended to avoid making direct social contacts with one another, presumably due to the high risks involved, as fighting can account for up to 7% of all fox mortalities. A revised model predicted that the rate of rabies spread would be slower than that predicted by the original one, and this effect was more pronounced at lower fox population densities. However, MAFF continues to employ the original, more pessimistic model as the basis of its contingency plans.

How efficient does fox control have to be to eliminate a rabies outbreak in Britain?

The original model was used to predict the spread of a rabies outbreak in the West Midlands conurbation. With no control, it was estimated that the disease would reach the edge of the conurbation within a year, and eradication of the disease would only be possible if almost 90% of the fox population was killed. Similar results were obtained for the three other urban areas (Bournemouth and Poole, Bristol, Leicester) that were investigated in detail using the model. However, once the more accurate data on fox contact rates were available, it was apparent that the same probability of successfully controlling the rabies outbreak could be achieved by a 5 to 15% lower level of fox control than predicted by the original model. This is not to say that it will be an easy task, only that with the same amount of effort there will be a greater chance of successfully containing and eradicating the disease within a specified control area than was originally thought.[88]

One factor to emerge from the revised model was the importance of the time of year of a rabies outbreak in determining successful control. The chance of success will be greatest if the disease is introduced in winter and lowest if it is introduced in spring. This may seem strange as fox contacts are highest in winter and so rabies will initially spread rapidly following an outbreak in winter. However, as the disease will start to spread from a single source, at the end of the winter the number

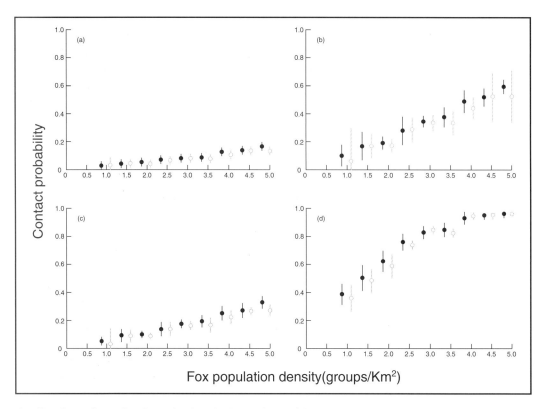

The effect of time of year of a rabies outbreak on the chance of successful control in Bristol under the original and revised versions of the model. Rabies was introduced at the beginning of (a) March – spring; (b) June – summer; (c) September – autumn and (d) December – winter. Original model in blue; revised model in black

of infected foxes will still be relatively small, and the onset of spring, the season with the fewest contacts, will considerably slow the rate of inter-group infection. By the end of the spring, there will still be few infected animals, so the chance of successful control will be increased. In contrast, for an outbreak that starts in the spring, the initial rate of inter-group infection will also be slow, but this will be followed by three seasons with more contacts before the damping effect of the spring season comes into play once more. Thus, there will be a greater opportunity for the infection to spread to more fox family groups, and the likelihood of successful control will be reduced. Unfortunately, the likelihood of introducing the disease to Britain is probably highest in the spring and summer, when more people travel abroad and hence the chance of smuggling an infected pet increases.

Can the required level of fox control be achieved?

The modelling studies show that if rabies were re-introduced into Britain it could in theory be contained and eradicated. However, the proposed control operation might be unsuccessful. To kill 90% of the foxes would require three poisoning campaigns with a 50% population reduction each time, four campaigns with a 40% reduction, five campaigns with a 30% reduction or eight campaigns with a 20% reduction. This has been attempted in a series of trials in Bristol using a biomarker rather than a poison in the bait, and with a density of baits twice that suggested in MAFF's urban rabies contingency plans. Only a third of the adult foxes and less than a quarter of the cubs or sub-adults ate the baits.[75] In an actual rabies epizootic, the baits will contain poison, and any fox eating a single bait will die, thus removing it from the population. As some foxes in the trial ate more than one bait with the biomarker, in a poisoning campaign a few more foxes are likely to find and eat a bait. However, this would not make a significant difference, and several baiting operations would be required.

Smith and Harris think that perhaps 85% would need to be killed to eradicate the disease in a programme of control lasting several months.[86] They concluded that attaining the very high levels of fox population control required in urban areas would be difficult. Killing such a number of foxes from an urban area has not been attempted anywhere to date.

One of the numerous practical problems of mounting a control operation is that the burying of baits is very labour-intensive, and thus many hundreds of people would be needed. Mounting such an operation will be difficult and spreading the available man-power too thinly is likely to reduce the chance of success. As the potential rate of spread of the disease in urban areas appears to be a little lower than first envisaged, it may be that in certain circumstances the control operation would be more effective if the control area was reduced so that a more concentrated effort could be achieved. This would only be applicable if it was certain that the risk was localized. So far this option has not been explored. A poisoning campaign in an urban area could be effectively supplemented by vaccine baits in the surrounding rural areas, which would have the advantage of acting as a back-up measure against the wider spread of the disease should any rabid animals disperse beyond the control zone.

How different are rural fox populations from those of urban areas?

Although the data on the demography, social organization, movement and contact behaviour of urban fox populations are now quite extensive,

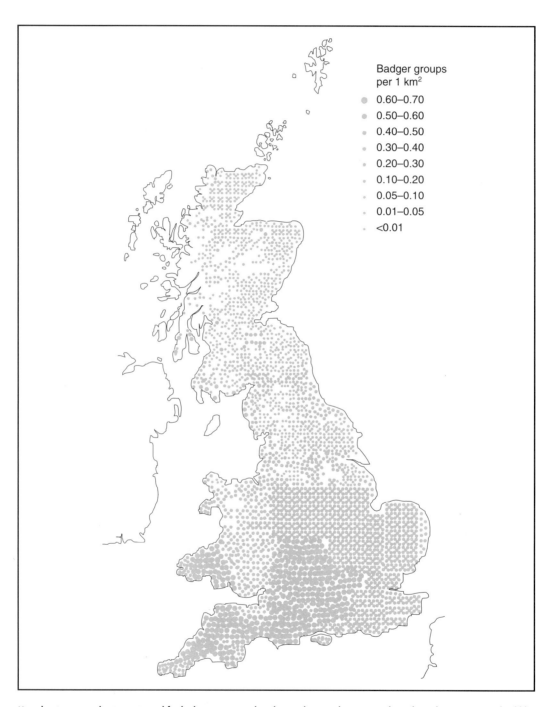

Map showing mean density estimated for badgers, measured as the number social groups per km², throughout Britain. It should be noted that the densities shown are the mean for each landscape type, and thus the actual densities in specific areas may be higher or lower than the respective means[92]

there is a lack of comparable information on rural fox populations, and so the contingency plans for rural areas are not based on a computer simulation model and are therefore less adaptable to specific circumstances. The most important first step towards improving our knowledge of rural fox populations would be to develop a means of predicting rural fox population densities from land use and habitat variables, in a similar way to that carried out for urban foxes.

Understanding the influence of the environment on fox contact behaviour is of great importance, as it will determine the relative significance of normal inter-group contacts and dispersal movements in spreading rabies in rural areas. An improved knowledge of the behaviour and organization of rural fox populations will be a major step forward in the development of rabies models and control strategies. Another potential problem in rural areas is the possibility of multiple hosts within the sylvatic disease cycle.

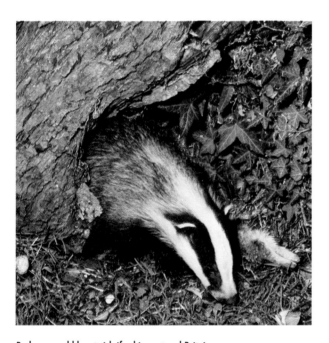

Badgers would be at risk if rabies entered Britain

Could any other species serve as a secondary host for the sylvatic disease cycle in Britain?

One feature of British fauna that sets it apart from mainland Europe, and which may be of some importance for rabies spread and control, is the extremely high density of badgers (*Meles meles*) in certain areas. In Europe, where badgers occur at much lower densities, they accounted for less than 1.5% of all rabies cases in 1993.[89] However, in Britain there are about 250 000 adult badgers, and these produce 175 000 cubs each year. This is more badgers than are found in any other mainland European country. In fact the badger population in Britain is very similar to the rural fox population – 207 000 adult foxes which produce about 365 000 cubs.[80] Moreover, the badger population is very unevenly distributed within Britain. Forty-seven per cent of all badgers occur in the south-west and south-east regions, which together make up just under a quarter of the total area of mainland Britain.[90] In these parts of Britain badger densities may locally exceed fox densities, and these are also the areas at the greatest risk of a rabies epidemic caused by a pet illegally brought across the English Channel. Whilst the most likely way in which a badger could transmit rabies to a human would be via a domestic dog, there have been reports of badgers attacking people.[91]

All the available evidence indicates that badgers are very much more common today than they were at the end of the nineteenth century, and as with foxes, the increase in badger numbers is thought to be mainly due to a decline in control brought about by fewer gamekeepers.[92] While foxes would be the main wildlife reservoir for the sylvatic form of the disease, were it to become endemic, in certain areas badgers might serve as a secondary reservoir of the disease. A substantial secondary reservoir, especially in a host which is at the centre of so much conservation interest, would make successful elimination of endemic rabies very difficult indeed.

What are the chances of successful eradication of rabies from Britain?

The computer simulations have highlighted the difficulties of controlling a rabies outbreak stemming from a single known point source of infection, even if control is started almost immediately. In reality, this may not be possible, especially if the source of infection is a smuggled pet. It is unlikely that owners would report breaking the law and, assuming that they recognize the signs, alert the authorities that a pet was rabid. Anticipating human behaviour in such an eventuality is difficult, but the owner might, for instance, drive off and abandon the pet some distance from home. This would mean that the source of infection might not be known and the first indication of the disease might not be the original rabid dog or cat, but the discovery of a rabid fox. This would raise immediately a number of questions:

• is this the first fox to become infected?

• did it become infected where it was found?

• is the focus of infection some distance away and has the animal moved to the point where it was found?

Even in continental Europe only a minority of rabid animals are located, and so in theory the disease could be present in Britain for some months before its presence was recognized. Another possibility is that there may be several point sources of infection, especially if the disease has become established and some infected foxes have dispersed from the area where the disease originated. There are many such possible scenarios, and any of them would considerably exacerbate the problems of controlling the epizootic, since the disease would have had a head start on the control measures. Although the problems of controlling a rabies outbreak in Britain are clear, there are at present no plans to deal with endemic disease.

The present outlook

The development of post-exposure treatment has meant that rabies is no longer a major threat to human life in developed countries. However, the significantly greater expense of attempting to control endemic disease, compared with maintaining a preventive strategy, is a convincing case for furthering research efforts into the means of successfully controlling the disease should it be re-introduced to Britain. The development of computer simulation models has given us a clear indication of the level of fox control that is required to eliminate rabies in these circumstances. Due to the extremely high densities of foxes in many urban areas, the level of control required is very high, and rates of bait uptake achieved in studies to date have been well below these target levels. For vaccination to become a successful strategy dramatic improvements in bait uptake would be necessary; the use of attractants to encourage foxes to take the baits may have a role to play. As the new estimates of contact rates between foxes in urban areas have led to revised estimates of the rate of disease spread, it is likely that concentrating the control effort into an area smaller than the 19 km radius currently favoured may increase the rate of bait uptake and hence the proportion of foxes reached by the poison. Using the models currently available it should be possible to determine the optimum size of the control area.

Given the low bait uptake rates that have so far been achieved, if rabies was introduced tomorrow into an urban area in a strain that could be both carried and transmitted by foxes, we cannot yet be certain that we can successfully control the disease within the designated control area, especially if the disease was introduced in the spring and summer into a city with a high population density of foxes. In such an eventuality, if the disease spread into the rural fox population, our current lack of knowledge of the social behaviour and organization of rural foxes would make it much more difficult to predict the pattern of further spread. The outlook for eradicating rabies once it was established within the fox population is not optimistic. Anderson *et al.* concluded that the government's contingency policy of killing foxes 'is unlikely to be effective once rabies becomes established within the fox population'.[93] Control efforts would be further complicated by the potential for badgers to act as secondary hosts in specific parts of the country.

Living with enzootic rabies in Britain

If MAFF's contingency plans for stopping the spread of a rabies outbreak in Britain failed, we would be faced with enzootic rabies in British wildlife; what would this mean in terms of our daily lives? Some critics of the system of quarantine argue that enzootic rabies is not such a 'bad thing', and that other countries, such as France and Germany, live with wildlife rabies. But we in Britain are used to the luxury of a generally benign nature: there are few poisonous snakes or insects and no man-eating wolves or bears or dangerous wild boars. Britons are used to relaxing in the countryside without fearing wildlife and feeling free to stroke stray cats and dogs in the streets. It is for this reason that the British public are the least prepared when they meet rabies abroad. Consequently a larger number of Britons contract the disease abroad than any other west European nationality.[94] Were rabies to become enzootic in this country, British people would have to curb their well-known friendliness towards most animals.

Children

Children are at particular risk from dog bites, presumably because of their lack of wariness of animals, small stature and their lesser ability to defend themselves. Furthermore, from the time of exposure, children develop rabies more quickly than adults. Every child would have to be taught to avoid contact with animals other than pets which were known to have been vaccinated.

It was estimated that 18 000 children under 16 years old attended accident and emergency departments for dog bites in 1992.[95] About 27 000 adults are also bitten by pets each year.[95] Many other cases are treated at home or by general practitioners. The total may be as high as 250 000 cases of dog bites in the UK each year.[96]

Anyone bitten by an unknown or sick animal or one whose vaccination history was uncertain or inadequate, would have to receive post-exposure treatment with rabies vaccination as soon as possible (Table 10, p. 112). Following treatment there is the inevitable waiting period to see whether symptoms appear. Patients may feel as if a death sentence is hanging over them and, considering the frequency of dog bites, the great anxiety which accompanies the long and variable incubation of rabies would become commonplace. Constant vigilance would be required.[11]

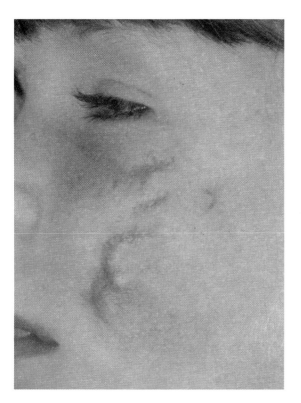

Child bitten by a dog

Ecological implications

Foxes and badgers are the main wildlife species which are likely to be affected should rabies become enzootic in Britain. Enzootic rabies would probably substantially reduce the populations of these species, and the effects might be particularly serious for badgers. In parts of the south-west, where the highest population densities occur, locally there may be around three groups of badgers per km^2, and a single group can have up to as many as 20 animals.[97] As these animals can share a single sett, this might be ideal for the transmission of the disease via aerosol infection, social grooming and fights with other members of the same group and members of neighbouring groups. Bite wounds, especially severe wounds, are probably more common in badgers than foxes.

Of other wild mammals in Britain, bats have already been discussed, and there is unlikely to be a significant involvement of other species. The only three carnivore species that are widespread and relatively common are mink (*Mustela vison*), stoats (*Mustela erminea*) and weasels (*Mustela nivalis*), but their population densities are not high and they are rarely involved in rabies cases in Europe. Squirrels (*Sciurus carolinenses*), like other rodents, have never been reported to initiate an epizootic and would become infected only as a result of spillover of rabies from other infected species.

The rarer carnivores – otters (*Lutra lutra*), pine martens (*Martes martes*), polecats (*Mustela putorius*) and the wildcat (*Felis sylvestris*) – are locally distributed at relatively low densities in the more remote areas, and since none feature prominently among wildlife rabies cases in Europe, they are also unlikely to be of importance in a rabies epizootic in Britain. However, pine martens can live close to humans in some areas, and so if one did become infected, it could pose a potential risk to humans locally.[98]

Chapter 7

Policy options for preventing rabies in Britain

It is a cliché that nothing in life is risk free. No system is entirely safe and this remains true for quarantine as well as for any system of vaccination, but what are the relative risks? Since July 1994 Britain has run a dual system of rabies control: quarantine for pets and vaccination and certification for certain commercially traded animals from within the European Union.

Before assessing the safety of quarantine as a system of rabies control, it is important to consider the risk of rabies entering a rabies-free nation without any such controls. However, although risk assessment is often presented as an exact science, interpretations may vary considerably depending on the factors included, and the weight given to those factors in the calculations.

In a report prepared for the European Commission by a sub-group of the Scientific Veterinary Committee, the risk of rabies entering a rabies-free member state from a rabies-infected member state was regarded as 'varying between small and negligible depending on the incidence of rabies in dogs in the infected state and on the volume of movement of dogs across the borders'; the risk from cats was considered similar.[99] According to the sub-group's calculations the risk of introducing rabies into a rabies-free country with no rabies controls would be as follows.

If 5000 dogs entered the UK from France every year, one would expect a dog incubating rabies to enter the UK once every 250 years. However, for a country with a higher incidence of rabies, such as Germany, the likelihood is increased significantly. If 5000 dogs a year travelled from Germany to Denmark a rabid dog would enter Denmark once every 31 years.

The sub-group emphasizes that the risk would be further reduced if the dog visited the rabies-free state for only a short period, such as the owner's holiday, and that these risks would be diminished further by precautions such as vaccination or quarantine. Yet there are other factors which raise the risks: first, the calculations include only numbers for dogs and exclude cats; second, they only consider one country at a time whereas animals are imported into rabies-free states from all nations in the EU, and third, the calculations rely on figures which may under-represent rabies incidence.

How effective is quarantine?

The risks presented by the UK system of quarantine can be assessed by examining its past record. Between 1922 and 1969 there were 27 cases of dogs and cats found incubating rabies in quarantine. Three of these cases died six months or later after first entering quarantine. One became rabid almost nine months after first entering quarantine and it is not known how it contracted the disease.[99] However, since vaccination on entry to quarantine was made compulsory (following the 1971 Waterhouse Committee's recommendation) two dogs have died without showing rabies symptoms but with rabies antigen in the brain and no animal has become rabid *after* release from quarantine. Thus quarantine without vaccination (until 1971) was at least 93.5% effective in detecting animals which were incubating the disease and quarantine regulations as they currently stand (with vaccination) have been 100% effective to date.

However, calculations have been made leading to the claim that, due to the variable incubation period of rabies, the probability of determining whether a dog has rabies under British quarantine may be lower than previously thought. The Infection Protection Unit of the Swedish Board of Agriculture estimates that there would be a mere 78% certainty of finding rabies in a dog during a six month period of quarantine and a nine and a half month period would be required for a 95% certainty.[64] Yet in practice, the British system of quarantine with its initial vaccination, has proved 100% reliable over more than 20 years. So, despite the variable incubation period for rabies, out of the approximately 200 000 cats and dogs vaccinated in quarantine, no known infected animal has been released.[100]

Although this is an impressive record, it could be argued that, as so few animals have died of rabies in quarantine, the risk of the disease entering the country is low, nevertheless any one of the 29 animals dying in quarantine might potentially have started a rabies outbreak. Since 1971 when vaccination was introduced on entry to quarantine, no further cases have occurred in kennels, apart from two animals who died from atypical rabies from live Flury vaccine administered before importation.[100] The latter cases point towards the efficacy of inactivated rabies vaccine for cats and dogs and the hazards of using obsolete live vaccines. It therefore appears that, although quarantine has been highly successful in controlling the risk of rabies entering Britain, this risk has proved a very small one.

Is quarantine cruel to animals?

The case has been put that unnecessary suffering is imposed on animals undergoing quarantine due to isolation from their owners. The pet may be psychologically damaged, away from familiar surroundings and 'abandoned' by its owner.[101] Animals are required to be detained for six months in a condition where they are segregated from their usual gregarious way of life. Contact with other animals should not occur, although pets of the same owner can be housed in the same cage, and their contact with humans is naturally reduced. Indications are that such contact is beneficial to the animal. Owners are allowed to visit, but an animal may be bewildered by the new circumstances and by the short visit of its owner. Some owners deliberately stay away so that the pets do not keep seeing them come and go without taking them with them. It has been suggested that some animals become so distressed that they refuse food and pine away. MAFF deny this, and certainly the statistics for animal deaths in quarantine do not suggest particularly high death rates. From 1990 to 1993 there were 36 001 dogs and cats in quarantine and less than 1.4% died, which is approximately the number of deaths in the outside pet population.

Animals' temperaments will change with their change in environment and living conditions vary considerably across the range of quarantine kennels. Exercise areas are limited and long walks not available, so their fitness may diminish under a restrictive regime. However, some kennels make every effort to have as much human contact as possible, thus minimizing the disruption to the animal. It may be all too easy to attribute human feelings to animals, and those in contact with dogs in quarantine suggest that most survive the experience well.

However, there may be room for improvement in the standards of quarantine facilities, both in construction and management. Quarantine kennels are licensed by MAFF. The licensing authorities are restricted by the legislation which allows them to control only certain specified items and leaves them unable to apply statutory standards for boarding. In the interim MAFF applies a Code of Practice.

The question of animals suffering through quarantine remains contentious. Is it, however, logical to consider a change of policy for the sake of the possible mild discomfort that a small minority of animals may experience at being removed from their owners for six months? Were rabies to break out in Britain, many animals might suffer agonizing rabies symptoms and die in great pain. Others might die from poisoning under MAFF's attempts to control an outbreak. While we may feel sentimental towards our own pet, and there may be room for improved quarantine standards, in this area a utilitarian approach seems more appropriate, safeguarding the greatest good for the greatest number.

Vaccination as a policy for rabies prevention

Open access of animals across the contiguous land borders of western European countries has long made quarantine an impracticable method of rabies control although it was applied until recently by a few European countries. Most have favoured vaccination as the only effective means of protecting their indigenous domestic animals. Many EU countries require dogs and cats to be vaccinated before entry is permitted.

For animals living in EU countries there is no coherent pattern of vaccination. For some it is compulsory countrywide, for others it is mandatory only for animals living in rabies-infected areas or in special circumstances. In France for example, vaccination is required for all dogs and cats living in the French administrative 'départements' (areas) infected with rabies, or for dogs and cats entering campsites and pet shows from any of the French departments. Horses in riding clubs in contaminated areas must be vaccinated; for other domestic species living in these areas vaccination is not required. For non-contaminated areas vaccination of dogs and cats is not mandatory but is recommended.

In Germany rabies vaccination of dogs and cats is not compulsory, but government authorities can impose local vaccination depending on prevailing epidemiological conditions. Most dog owners vaccinate their pets voluntarily as this allows freedom of movement in rabies-infected areas. In case of contact with a rabid animal the vaccinated dog can be put under observation and not destroyed. In Italy it would appear that much the same applies; vaccination is compulsory for all animals in at-risk areas, on entry to Italy and if taken abroad.

Norway and Sweden: a change of policy

Although dogs have become rabid in France, experimentally the European fox-adapted rabies virus is less readily transmitted to other species than between foxes. It has never been shown that cats and dogs have spread the fox-adapted virus into new areas or initiated new epizootics.[102] On this basis Norway and Sweden have decided that vaccination and antibody testing will be sufficient to maintain their rabies-free status when applied to dogs and cats imported from EU and EFTA (European Free Trade Association) regions where foxes are the main vectors. This does not apply to imports from other countries.

Prior to May 1994, Norway and Sweden required quarantine for all dogs and cats coming from rabies-infected countries, including 'potentially rabies-infected countries', i.e. countries where no cases of rabies had been reported for several years but where dogs and cats could be imported without quarantine. After consultation with an expert group, the Norwegian and Swedish veterinary authorities decided that quarantine should no longer be required for dogs and cats imported from the EU/EFTA countries and from the territory of Svalbard.

Rabies vaccination followed by determination of antibody titre now replace the former quarantine requirement for dogs and cats imported from the EU/EFTA. Dogs must be at least three months old and cats 14 months old when first vaccinated. They must have serum antibody levels of at least 0.5 IU/ml, measured by the rapid fluorescent focus inhibition test (RFFIT) (Appendix III), before they are eligible for movement into and out of Sweden. The permit issued for movement is valid for one year. During the movement outside of Sweden the animal must not visit non-EU/EFTA countries.[103]

Animals imported without quarantine from the EU/EFTA must have resided in the EU/EFTA at least one year before entry/re-entry to Norway or Sweden. Quarantine is still required for carnivore species other than dogs and cats – and for dogs and cats imported from countries other than the EU/EFTA countries.[104] The long period (14 months) before cats can be vaccinated is a reflection of the less well known effect of rabies vaccination in cats. It is likely that this period will be reduced when cat responses have been analysed.

Difficulties encountered with Norway and Sweden's policy change

The main problem encountered within the first six months of the policy change has been the low antibody levels observed in animals following their first dose of vaccine. Vaccination against rabies is prohibited in

Norway and Sweden, except for the purpose of travelling to a rabies-infected country. Therefore, the majority of the dog population is unvaccinated and almost 20% of these animals show antibody levels lower than 0.5 IU/ml four months after their first vaccination. In comparison, adult dogs imported to Norway after several annual rabies vaccinations often had high titres (above 2–3 IU/ml). Booster vaccination one month after the first vaccination for animals that have never previously been vaccinated against rabies is now recommended in Norway and Sweden.[104]

The figures for Sweden are the responses to vaccinations in a country which formerly forbade vaccination of cats and dogs. The figures for Germany are the responses to vaccination in a country where vaccination was compulsory in certain rabies-endemic areas. Table 7a and b shows that a single vaccination is not always sufficient to enable an animal to pass the blood test since only 72% of nearly 2 000 animals had over 0.5 IU/ml antibody in their sera. It is not possible from these figures to determine the actual percentage of animals that would have passed the test after re-vaccination, as the histories of those dogs vaccinated 1.7.94–30.9.94 have still to be catalogued and some may have received one vaccination only. An alternative to the vaccination schedule may be

Table 7 Analysis of rabies neutralizing antibody (IU/ml) in (a) dog and (b) cat sera measured by rapid fluorescent focus inhibition test (RFFIT)

(a) Import date	01.01.94–30.06.94			01.07.94–30.09.94		
Antibody titre	$n > 0.5$ IU	$n < 0.5$ IU	$\% > 0.5$ IU	$n > 0.5$ IU	$n < 0.5$ IU	$\% > 0.5$ IU
Denmark	503	24	95	246	3	99
Sweden	935	635	59	794	186	82
Germany	351	51	87	48	5	90
Total	1789	710	72	1088	194	84
(b) Import date	01.01.94–30.06.94			01.07.94–30.09.94		
Antibody titre	$n > 0.5$ IU	$n < 0.5$ IU.	$\% > 0.5$ IU	$n > 0.5$ IU	$n < 0.5$ IU	$\% > 0.5$ IU
Denmark	31	0	100	11	1	92
Sweden	109	7	94	52	0	100
Germany	16	3	84	4	0	100
Total	156	10	96	67	1	98

to test the blood and re-vaccinate three months after the first vaccination, if the titre is too low, followed by a second blood test one month later. This would ensure a higher percentage, if not all, of animals passing the test and an increased level of protection with longer duration for all vaccinated animals.

Should Britain replace quarantine with a policy of vaccination, certification and identification?

Most western European countries, where fox rabies has been the only reservoir, see quarantine as an unnecessary hindrance to trade and movement. They regard vaccination and antibody testing as a suitable alternative.[105] The spectacular advances in rabies control, particularly the progress toward the eradication of the wildlife reservoirs by oral vaccination in western Europe, probably justify a re-examination of Britain's present regulations.

The report of the Commons Select Committee on Agriculture recommended that a system of vaccination and certification should replace quarantine for pet animals entering Britain from EU member states and 'approved' rabies-free countries with immediate effect, though no mechanism for granting approval to these 'rabies-free' countries is described.[61]

The wider case for abandoning quarantine and substituting vaccine certificates of immune status for dogs and cats is supported by impressive evidence assembled by Aubert.[106,107] However, some aspects of this evidence may not convince all observers. There is more information about canine vaccination than there is for cats. It is noted that 'responses may vary and be poor both among individuals and in some breeding conditions'. King observes that animals vaccinated while incubating the disease may develop antibodies without the progression of the disease being affected.[100] Successful vaccination of every dog and cat cannot be guaranteed.

Vaccination may fail if:

- the animal is vaccinated when too young
- the animal is incubating rabies at the time of vaccination (there is no reliable test able to detect the presence of the rabies virus in a living animal during the incubation period)
- the vaccinated animal is immunocompromised.

Most of these pitfalls can be overcome by the use of accurate serological testing. Were serological testing allowed at the point of import (i.e. a British port) the safeguards would be secure. If serological testing is carried out in the exporting country, the importing country must rely on certification. There is considerable incentive to falsify as quarantine fees are high, added to which is the inconvenience and upset of separation from a pet for six months or having to leave the animal at home. Where there is insufficient confidence in the test results or certification which accompany the animal, confirmatory antibody tests could be carried out at the port of entry. This would not only help to apprehend those animals dispatched with inaccurate documentation, but the presence of checking procedures could also act as a deterrent against falsification. However both practical and scientific difficulties remain in serological testing.

Serological testing

Although rabies neutralizing antibody is not the only component concerned in the immune response, it is associated with the immunity induced by rabies vaccine. The mouse neutralization test (MNT) (Appendix III) is being replaced by the more reliable rapid fluorescent focus inhibition test (RFFIT).[108] Although expensive, the RFFIT is considered the most reliable method and it avoids the use of live animals, but criticisms continue of both the consistency of its results and the practicalities of carrying out large numbers of such tests.[109]

Nevertheless, work is continuing to ensure that RFFIT results are consistent. In an experiment involving international laboratory co-operation, a panel of dog sera was tested against a known reference serum from the Office International des Epizooties (Nancy) laboratory at nine other laboratories; the results from eight of the laboratories were within the expected range, but those of one were not.[110] International agreement is needed among national serological testing laboratories on reference sera of a specified potency to enable standardization of tests.

Practical difficulties with RFFIT

A laboratory capable of carrying out RFFIT requires high cost technology which can safely handle live rabies virus, and to ensure accuracy and consistency, needs to test many sera each day. At present, the UK lacks such a facility. Given the many British owners who may wish to take part in a vaccination and certification scheme, were one introduced, such a facility would be required to allow the animals to comply with the British regulations on their return.

Were such a scheme introduced, a large increase in the number of animals travelling into Britain is expected, as many pets would be taken on holidays. Estimates are difficult to make as MAFF does not collect statistics on the countries of export of animals entering British quarantine, so we do not know how many of those animals passing through quarantine would be eligible for a scheme of vaccination, certification and identification. Furthermore, if on inspection at the port of entry there was doubt about the accuracy of an animal's health records or its identification, it might be necessary to carry out a repeat antibody test while the animal awaited entry into Britain. Facilities would then be required to hold the animal in isolation at the port while the test was done.

To safeguard against testing errors, the WHO recommends that two positive serological test results should be achieved before an animal be allowed entry to a rabies-free country.[111] However, the system recommended by the Commons Select Committee on Agriculture does not call for such a safeguard.[61] This raises particular concern as many rabies-free countries outside Europe do not have RFFIT or comparable testing facilities. Under the scheme recommended by the Commons Select Committee, these countries would be eligible to import the pet animals into Britain without quarantine. For assurance that animals had sufficient antibody responses to rabies vaccines from countries whose facilities were not deemed adequate to provide accurate test results, further testing would be necessary in the UK.

Practical obstacles to policies of vaccination

Most of the difficulties in successfully implementing a policy of vaccination, certification and identification lie in logistics. Most important of all is certification and identification of the immigrant animal, which is fraught with difficulties. The WHO's International Vaccination Certificate for dogs and cats lists species, age, sex, breed, colour and coat markings among the criteria for identifying individual animals. However, it is not infrequently the case that even species and sex cannot be accepted with confidence. As some authorities have difficulty in distinguishing which species of dogs are covered by the Dangerous Dogs Act 1991, the remaining physical characteristics might be less certain as identifying marks and the WHO draws attention to the hazards of misidentification of animals from vaccination certificates.

This really leaves only microchip implants and, to a lesser extent, ear tattoos as 'fool' or evasion proof means of matching, with any certainty, an animal with its vaccination certificate. There is space for recording booster doses of vaccine on the WHO certificate, how frequently this is required depends much on the type of vaccine and the route by which it was administered. A new certificate would no doubt indicate the animal's immune status in international units of antibody at the proposed time of entry and authenticated by the laboratory responsible for the test. Ear tattoos are difficult to inscribe legibly, and may be 'doctored' relatively easily. Microchip implants appear to be the most satisfactory form of identification although the problem of incompatible technology must be overcome.

Microchip identification

In all concerns regarding responsible pet ownership, identification is a key to allowing satisfactory management procedures together with the benefit of returning lost pets to owners. The advent of the Balai Directive in July 1994 has meant that EU cats and dogs entering Britain as commercially traded animals now require microchip identification.[25,112] The Dangerous Dogs Act 1991 also required microchip implants for dogs specified under Section 1 to be placed on the Index of Exempted Dogs.

Where paperwork is an important part of a compliance system of control, the inevitability of forgery must be considered. The accuracy of the animal's identity – whether it has been replaced by another animal, or had its blood sample replaced – for examination purposes must be without question. The reliability of vaccine application must also be verifiable over a world market. Many millions of pounds are involved in vaccination programmes. It is therefore essential that accuracy, reliability and easy recoverability of permanent identification should be used. A technical specification allowing compatibility between microchips and their readers (without specifying manufacturers) should also be agreed. None of these requirements need exclude a variety of chip, reader or register usages.

It is essential that compatibility allows inter-country use for adequate control measures. Additional relevant information, such as type of vaccine used, batch number, results of antibody titre tests, name of verifiable veterinarian involved in treatment, date of vaccination, date on which vaccination renewal is due, countries visited, and any necessary precautions due to known medical history may be retrievable using a unique identification number. It has been suggested that the initial use of mandatory microchip implants in traded animals, following the Balai Directive, has missed an opportunity to provide the fullest information in a readily retrievable store by neglecting the retention of relevant data beyond the point of arrival. History has shown that there is a reasonable need for caution in knowing where and when animals originated when a disease outbreak occurs. It would seem sensible to record animals with microchips on a central register so that information could be retrieved should it become necessary. The ANIMO system could act as such a register.

The ANIMO system

At present, when livestock or a cat or dog exported under the Balai Directive is to be moved from other EU member states into Britain, the veterinary authorities in the country of origin must give advance notice to MAFF of the animals' time of arrival, point of entry to the UK, final destination and route.[25] This information is passed through the ANIMO (ANImal MOvements) computer system and stored by MAFF. Also included in the data are the animal's health certificate number, the date of the certificate and the name of the veterinary surgeon who signed it. However, for animals imported under the Balai Directive, there is no provision for including the identification number of their microchip implants. The information carried on the microchip would help to identify the animal. Were an outbreak of rabies to occur or be suspected, this information would be useful in tracing the animal and its movements and discovering the origin of any forgery of certification.

The format of information to be passed through the ANIMO system is decided by the European Commission, because it requires agreement between all EU countries exporting animals within the Union. In order to ensure that animals transported under the Balai Directive can be securely identified at all times, the European Commission should specify that the unique identifying number of the microchip implant be included in information transferred by ANIMO. Such a requirement could also be used for pet dogs and cats entering Britain were a system of vaccination, certification and identification to be introduced.

The Balai Directive[25]

Most of the concerns raised by the implementation of the Balai Directive are those affecting policies of vaccination and certification generally. The safeguards of the system stipulated by MAFF appear stronger than those recommended by the Commons Select Committee on Agriculture, specifying that all animals imported under its regulations will be examined within 48 hours of arrival at the premises of destination by the local Divisional Veterinary Officer who will check the certification, read

MODEL
HEALTH CERTIFICATE[a]
(to be accompanied by the animals' vaccination certificates)

for placing on the market in the United Kingdom and Ireland of dogs and cats not originating in those countries

DOGS/CATS[b,c]

Consignor Member State . . . .

I   Number of animals . . . .

II Identification of animals . . . .

Number of animals	Species/ breed	Age, or date of birth	Sex	Colour	Type and marking of coat	Number encoded in implanted transponder

(Use continuation sheet if necessary.)

III Origin of the animals

Address of the registered holding . . . .

. . . .

IV Destination of the animals

The animals will be sent

from . . . .
(place)

to . . . .
(place of destination)

by[d] rail, road, aircraft, boat/ship[b] . . . .

Name and address of consignor . . . .

Name and address of consignee . . . .

V   Health information

I, the undersigned, certify that the animal(s) described above meet the following requirements.

(a) They have been examined today and show no clinical sign of disease.

(b) They have been vaccinated against rabies for at least six months and, additionally, in the case of dogs, against canine distemper.

(c) They have undergone, between the first and third months after primary vaccination or a re-vaccination against rabies, a serological test showing a protective antibody titre of at least 0.5 international units. This serological test was carried out in accordance with the World Health Organization specifications.

(d) The owner or person responsible for the registered holding has provided me with a signed statement to the effect that:

the animal/s was/were[b] born on the registered holding and has/have[b] remained there since birth, with no contact with any wild animal susceptible to rabies.

VI This certificate is valid for ten days from the date of examination.

Done at . . . .**on** . . . .
(date of examination)

Stamp

. . . .
(signature of official veterinarian or veterinarian responsible for the holding of origin and empowered for this purpose by the competent authority)

NOTES

[a] Health certificates may be drawn up only for animals which are to be transported in the same mode of transport and which come from the same holding and which are being sent to the same consignee.

[b] Delete where not applicable.

[c] The certificate is valid for only one species at a time.

[d] Give the registration number in the case of lorries, trucks, vans or cars, the flight number in the case of aircraft, the name in the case of boat/ship, and in the case of rail travel, the estimated date and time of arrival

A health certificate for commercially traded cats and dogs entering Britain

the implanted microchip and possibly take a second blood sample to confirm the titre of the antibody against rabies.

Not only are the Balai Directive's requirements, as implemented by MAFF, reassuringly strict, but the animals pose a lower risk than pets, as they have never moved from the premises on which they were born (except possibly to attend a veterinary practice for treatment under restraint), have avoided contact with wild animals and are so few in number. Until February 1995 only two cats and three dogs had passed through the system and one animal was refused entry due to failure to comply with the requirements.

There are grounds for believing that the system recommended by the Commons Select Committee on Agriculture could not be implemented immediately, as the Committee suggests, without increasing the risk to Britain's rabies-free status. There are many difficulties both practical and technical which must first be overcome.

Chapter 8

Financial implications of various rabies policies[*]

It is difficult to calculate precisely the real financial costs of the various rabies policies when there are so many unknown variables involved, but some broad estimates may nonetheless be useful to gain an idea of where expenditure would arise. The four cases for comparison are:

1 a situation of enzootic rabies in Britain with no attempt to eradicate the disease from wildlife

2 retaining Britain's rabies-free status through the current system of quarantine

3 replacing quarantine with a system of vaccination, certification and identification

4 attempting the eradication of rabies from Britain were it to become enzootic.

Costs of enzootic rabies in Britain

Research and the enforcement of measures to prevent rabies returning to Britain are expensive but this cost is insignificant compared with the cost of a control programme to safeguard public health and that of domestic animals were rabies to become enzootic. Essential measures would include the vaccination of domestic animals, prophylactic measures for people at risk and post-exposure treatment for people who may have been exposed to the virus. The annual cost of rabies prevention and research in Britain is currently about £750 000.[70]

Were no attempts made to prevent the spread of rabies in Britain (and therefore no resources spent carrying out contingency plans) initial costs following an outbreak of rabies would include the compensation of farmers for the deaths of their livestock (around 7% of the rabies cases in Europe in 1993 occurred among cattle bitten by rabid foxes).[89] Vaccination of all pets susceptible to rabies would be necessary with repeat vaccinations annually (see Table 8).

[*] All costings at 1995 prices unless referenced otherwise.

Table 8 Financial implications of four rabies policies and scenarios*

Rabies remaining at large	
Item	**Cost**
Pre-exposure vaccination of HDCV rabies vaccine in humans at basic NHS price	£54.75 (3 doses) (or one-tenth of this dose can safely be used intradermally)
Boosters after exposure for those vaccinated	£36.50 (2 doses)
Post-exposure vaccination of HDCV rabies vaccine in humans	£109.50 (6 doses) of the vaccine
UK immunoglobulin at 40 pence per IU (given with vaccine as part of post-exposure treatment)	about £400–£600 per patient (depending on weight)
Rabies vaccine for animals (dose requirement varies per species but, for dogs and cats only one dose is initially required followed by an annual booster dose)	£25 annual total for vaccine and veterinary consultation fee for cat or dog
For all dogs (6.65 million) in Britain to be vaccinated annually	£166.25 million
For all cats (7.18 million) in Britain to be vaccinated annually	£179.5 million
Retaining Britain's rabies-free status through use of quarantine system	
Cost to pet owners	£10 million annual quarantine fees (1994)
Cost to taxpayer of rabies prevention and research	approximately £0.75 million (1993)
Replacing quarantine with vaccination and identification	
Cost to pet owners – vaccination	£25 annual total for vaccine and veterinary consultation fee for cat or dog; a further £25 if booster vaccination required for the animal to reach the antibody titre
Cost to pet owners – serological test	£35 for one tissue culture RFFIT (rapid fluorescent focus inhibition test); two may be required
Cost to pet owners – microchip implant (identification)	£10 for microchip, fitting and computerization of animal health records for life
If rabies did enter Britain accidentally, how much would it cost to eradicate the disease once more?	
Estimated costs in France of rabies control programme	£20 million annually (1993)

* All costings at 1995 prices unless stated otherwise

The cost to the NHS of rabies would be significant. This would include maintaining stocks of human vaccine and immunoglobulin for any case of an animal bite. A person bitten by an unknown animal, or one whose vaccination history was uncertain or inadequate, would have to receive post-exposure treatment including rabies vaccination as soon as possible. The cost of treating a single human exposed to rabies or suspected rabies stands at somewhere between £480 and £680 for the pharmaceuticals alone, not including professional time. Pre-exposure prophylaxis would be required by all those involved in work with animals: veterinary surgeons, local authority animal health inspectors and dog wardens, those working in dog kennels and catteries, zoo and park personnel, pet shop staff, the police and circus performers – not an insignificant number. In 1989 it was reported that the US expenditure associated with post-bite treatment was approximately $230 million annually, in a country where human rabies rarely occurs.[113]

Although human deaths from rabies are extremely rare in developed countries where safe and effective human anti-rabies vaccines are available, the treatment cost in intensive care of those few people who would inevitably contract the disease in a rabies endemic country, is extremely high: the average daily in-patient cost of being in an intensive

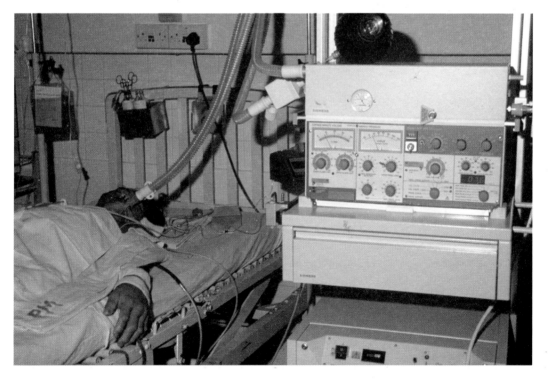

An intensive care unit

care unit is £658 (figures for Scotland, 1994). Furthermore, such treatment is likely to put out of use an urgently needed intensive care unit for some time to allow for disinfection. Cundy recommends, in addition, the provision of isolation facilities in UK intensive care units for rabies victims.[114] Advice to physicians on the care of patients with rabies is provided in the Department of Health and Social Security & Welsh Office's *Memorandum on Rabies*, 1977, and the eighth report of the WHO's Expert Committee on Rabies.[18,111]

The British public are also likely to be less aware of the dangers of rabies than inhabitants of rabies-enzootic countries. Animals suffering from the disease may not be diagnosed and animal bites could go untreated. Even in the US where rabies is enzootic among wildlife and medicine highly advanced, human rabies is often unsuspected in its victims.

The cost of quarantine

Quarantine costs around £1200 for a dog and around £1000 for a cat.[115] This is expensive compared with the costs of vaccination and sadly causes some pets to be left behind when a family emigrates. Based on an average of 5550 dogs and 3450 cats put through British quarantine each year, pet owners pay £10 110 000 annually in quarantine fees.

Costs of a system of vaccination, certification and identification

The UK veterinary price of rabies vaccine per vial/dose for animals is £7.19.[116] This is given initially with an annual booster of the same dose at the same cost. The pet owner pays the vet approximately £25. With an additional cost of £10 for a microchip, its fitting and the computerization of records, together with two blood tests at £35 each, the total is £105 or £70 if only one test were necessary. If a second (booster) vaccination were necessary, as has been the case in the majority of dogs vaccinated for travel in Sweden and Norway, the total cost could be £130.

Were a system of vaccination, certification and identification introduced in Britain for animals from the EU and perhaps also those from rabies-free countries, quarantine would remain necessary for animals imported from rabies-endemic areas outside the EU. The question has been raised whether the currently independent quarantine kennels would remain economically viable with only half their present income, possibly making it necessary for government to subsidize the quarantine kennel industry to ensure its survival.

Costs of eradication

The economic implications of enzootic rabies in Britain would depend on how great an attempt was made to stamp out the disease. Vaccination of wildlife is costly, and it is questionable whether this would prove an effective form of control in Britain. Killing many rabies susceptible animals could prove untenable due to public hostility. Although no figures are available for a sustained programme aimed at eradicating rabies from British wildlife, the annual expenditure on rabies control in France is estimated at £20 million.[70]

Chapter 9

Reviewing the issues

The risk of rabies entering Britain

In Chapter Seven the risks of importing rabies into Britain from another European nation are discussed using evidence prepared by bodies considering the replacement of quarantine with a system of vaccination. An average of 5500 dogs passed through British quarantine each year between 1990 and 1993 and many more dogs and cats would enter Britain if such a scheme of vaccination, certification and identification was introduced. Finland experienced a ten-fold increase in animal imports following the replacement of quarantine with a similar scheme. It was estimated that with no import controls (i.e. without vaccination and accompanying checks), one rabies-infected dog could be expected to enter the country every 23 years; it is worth noting that the infected animal may equally arrive in the first year as in the twenty-third.[117] However, were a system of vaccination with identification and serological testing to be introduced, the risk would be much lower. Dogs would only enter the country without vaccination or with inadequate vaccination as the result of failures in the system, through error, attempted fraud, or smuggling.

Figures arrived at by the Scientific Veterinary Committee of the European Commission state that if 5000 dogs were imported from Germany into Britain each year (the EU nation with the highest incidence of rabies) without any import controls such as vaccination, only one animal every 31 years could be expected to be incubating rabies.[99] However, these figures rely on *reported* cases of rabies in dogs which may well under-represent the true numbers affected, and cats are not considered at all (an average of 3450 cats entered Britain legally each year between 1990 and 1993). Furthermore, such figures ignore the significance of importing a single case of an infectious disease: one case introduced into a susceptible population may be enough to start an animal epidemic (epizootic), with potentially devastating effects.

In conclusion, there are several flaws to the calculations which form the basis of recent ECC policy changes. Not only may rabies be more prevalent among dogs and cats in Europe than represented by the available figures, but any single rabid animal entering Britain might destroy Britain's rabies-free status forever. If a pet cat or dog could transmit the European fox-adapted rabies virus into the British fox population, the consequences could be devastating. Furthermore, a high level of smuggling may weaken the impact of measures taken within the law to prevent the spread of rabies.

Rabies in Europe

Although obtaining accurate figures on the incidence of rabies in wildlife is fraught with difficulties, it is clear that the European oral fox vaccination programme is succeeding; rabies is being eradicated from European foxes and consequently from surrounding wildlife. From 1989 to 1992 the number of rabid wild animals reported in Europe fell by more than 50%.[51] In France and Germany in particular the decrease has been even more dramatic: between 1989 and 1993 the total numbers of rabid animals reported to the WHO in France and Germany decreased by 90%. However, complete eradication has not yet been achieved, with 1045 reported cases of rabid animals in western Europe and 2926 cases in eastern Europe in the first six months of 1994 and during the same period Germany suffered a setback with a significant rise in reported rabies cases.[118] It has been hypothesized that, were rabies eradicated from the fox population, the fox's place as primary vector of rabies might be taken by another species, such as the raccoon dog. However, encouraging developments continue in the field of oral animal vaccines, which in such an event, might lead to the eradication of rabies from new vector species.

If rabies entered Britain, its most likely route would be via a cat or dog that had been bitten by a rabid fox. The controversy continues as to whether a dog or cat carrying European fox-adapted rabies would merely act as the 'end host' of the virus, or whether it would be capable of starting an epizootic among animals, particularly foxes, in Britain. Sweden and Norway have based their change of policy on the evidence suggesting that fox-adapted rabies, if carried by dogs and cats, is unlikely to establish epizootics in other species. However, the controversy over this question continues.

It is sometimes assumed that because rabies was successfully eradicated in 1902 and 1922 and if rabies can be eradicated from Europe, which remains to be seen, then any outbreak in Britain could also be halted successfully. In both of Britain's past outbreaks of rabies, the main vectors and infected animals were dogs, which as companion animals, are easier to control than wildlife. The spread of rabies was therefore prevented by relatively simple precautions such as muzzling, enabling the disease to die out.

Today, however, the British animal population differs significantly from both earlier this century, when the fox population was smaller and sparser, and from the rest of Europe today. Britain's urban fox population has the highest density of any European country and this factor makes a policy of oral vaccination less likely to succeed, as a higher proportion of foxes would need to develop immunity to break the cycle of infection. Research suggests that if rabies were to become established in British wildlife, its eradication might prove extremely difficult. To stamp out rabies, even the culling of many foxes would not guarantee success, and the toll on Britain's wildlife would be considerable. Poisoning foxes with strychnine is the method outlined in MAFF's current contingency plans for the outbreak of rabies, and there is a risk that animals other than the fox would suffer an unpleasant death by strychnine poisoning.

Rabies and the threat to human life

Around the world rabies causes many deaths and great suffering. Twenty-five thousand or more human rabies deaths a year occur in India alone. Europe has been more fortunate: not only are relatively painless vaccines which rarely cause side-effects available for humans, but the vector by which rabies spreads also lessens the threat to humans; in much of Asia and Africa dogs are the main vectors of rabies and their close relationship with man brings a far higher transmission rate than the wildlife rabies prevalent in Europe.

For western Europeans, rabies poses a limited danger to public health, but the nature of the disease means that ensuring public safety is costly. For the human post-exposure treatment to work it is essential that those suspected of exposure to the virus receive vaccination promptly, preferably within the first 24 hours. Considerable resources are therefore involved in ensuring its ready availability across rabies-infected countries.

It must be accepted that however advanced the medical care available, if rabies is present, a small number of individuals may die. To seek treatment following exposure to rabies requires awareness of an event in which transmission could have occurred – a bite or scratch, for instance. Since

1960 more than 20% of rabies patients in the USA (12 out of 51 cases) were not aware of any exposure to a rabid animal and therefore they had no reason to seek anti-rabies vaccination.[119] Unfortunately, once symptoms have appeared, little can be done to prevent death.

The Channel Tunnel

Britain's island status has greatly aided retention of rabies-free status since 1922, but with the channel tunnel, Britain is now permanently linked to continental Europe. These two facts have caused widespread concern that rabid animals will travel through the tunnel into Britain. However, the tunnel's in-built safeguards and an understanding of rabies in France provide great reassurance.

Only limited areas of France are affected by rabies, and in recent years the disease has not been found within 100 miles of the French tunnel mouth. Additionally, the precautions set in place for keeping animals out of the tunnels are extremely comprehensive. Not only would it be unlikely for an animal to enter the tunnel in the first instance, due to the three sets of barriers at the French tunnel mouth and the disturbing noises and lights, but once inside, it would face a journey of 31 miles with the likelihood of being killed by the passage of high-speed trains, only to encounter three similar sets of barriers at the British end of the tunnel. Although rodents may be small enough to survive the onslaught of the high velocity trains, they have never been known to initiate an epizootic of rabies. Furthermore, the trains travelling through the tunnel are hermetically sealed and so unable to deposit any waste or fodder which could encourage the survival of animals. The safeguards of the channel tunnel therefore do not suggest that its presence increases the risk of rabies entering Britain.

The European Union

As previously stated, it is Britain's physical separation from continental Europe which has allowed the eradication and maintenance of freedom from many of the major veterinary diseases, not least rabies, which affect other parts of Europe. It is this insularity which clashes with the aims of the European Union as enshrined in the Treaty Establishing the European Community (formerly known as the Treaty of Rome): the promotion of the free movement of goods, services, people and capital between the member nations.

The European Commission aims to eradicate diseases which make necessary such measures as quarantine which impede movement within the EU. While pursuing the harmonization of the rules governing the movement of goods and people within the EU, the European Commission has also funded the vaccination of foxes aimed at eradicating terrestrial rabies from Europe.

Before the advent of the single European market in January 1993, quarantine was used for all livestock entering Britain. However, since then, while Britain has retained its role in keeping rabies out of Britain through its policy of quarantine for pets, the responsibility for the health standards of livestock has been transferred to the exporting countries. There is some evidence that since this transfer, the movement of disease between countries has also increased, as in the import of warble fly in cattle from France.

The Treaty of Rome allows member states to prevent free entry across their borders of certain goods on the grounds of protecting the public health and it is under such a provision that Britain has been able to retain its quarantine regulations.[44] It is therefore the case that border checks aimed at keeping rabies out of Britain, so long as they conform to the principles of proportionality and non-discrimination, should continue to be lawful.

The role of public health in EU legislation has been strengthened by the Maastricht Treaty (Article 129) which gives the Union a remit for public health. Thus, in drafting EU legislation, the Commission will have a responsibility towards improved public health, as well as promoting free trade and movement within the Union. Both of these factors should assist Britain in safeguarding its health standards in the future.

The consequences of rabies becoming endemic in Britain

Changes to the British way of life following the spread of endemic rabies in Britain would be far reaching. All pets would require vaccination; everyone involved in work with animals would need to be vaccinated; and any bite or scratch from a sick animal or an animal of unknown or inadequate vaccination history would have to be treated immediately. There would follow the agonizing wait of the long and variable incubation period to see whether rabies developed. Children, who are particularly susceptible to dog bites, would need to be warned from a young age of the necessity for reporting such incidents. Every child would have to be taught to avoid animals other than pets which were known to have been vaccinated. The well known British affection for animals would have to be tempered by caution; no longer could people stroke passing dogs or cats in the street and contact with wildlife would require even greater caution.

The economic implications of endemic rabies in Britain would depend on how great an attempt was made to stamp out the disease, and how successful attempts proved to be. The NHS budget for pharmaceuticals, already overstretched, would have to meet the cost of supplying anti-rabies vaccine and immunoglobulin across the entire country for immediate treatment of those exposed or suspectedly exposed to the virus. It is therefore widely agreed that the most appropriate policy is to keep rabies out of Britain. Which policies would succeed in doing so remain under debate.

The current system – advantages and disadvantages of quarantine

The overriding and widely accepted benefit of quarantine is its impressive record of success. Since 1971, when vaccination on arrival was introduced to animals' six months' stay in quarantine, not a single infected animal has been released; between 1971 and 1992 200 000 cats and dogs passed through quarantine.[100] However, while its success rate since 1971 could be said to be 100%, only two animals have actually died of rabies in quarantine. It could also be said to contribute positively in a small way to Britain's balance of payments, bringing as it does, revenue from abroad. However, on the minus side, quarantine is expensive for owners, impedes the free movement of people between nations and separates loved pets from their owners for a considerable length of time. People reliant on guidedogs and 'hearing dogs' (which alert their owners to sounds such as doorbells and alarm clocks) may be prevented from travelling abroad. Is there a safe system which could offer equal protection from rabies but without these costs? To make a full assessment, we must consider the alternative: certified vaccination of animals with confirmation of effectiveness by serological testing.

The alternative – vaccination and identification with serological testing

Systems of vaccination and identification differ from country to country. It is assumed that if a system were introduced into Britain it would follow the recommendations of the Commons Select Committee on Agriculture.[61] Legislation following the Balai Directive has already enabled traded

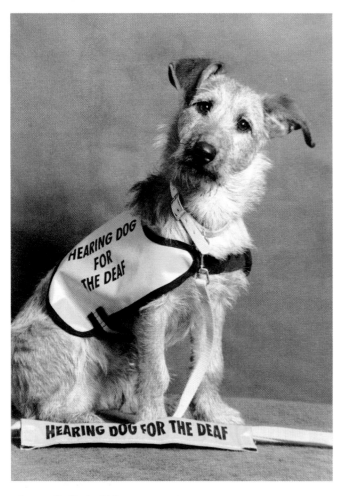

A hearing dog for the deaf

animals which have been vaccinated to enter Britain without quarantine under certain circumstances, but the numbers involved, and therefore the risk presented, are at present extremely small.[25]

Vaccination has been known to fail to protect animals fully from challenges with the rabies virus; in practice this has occurred if the recently vaccinated animal has been bitten by a rabid fox and proceeds to develop the disease. In France, vaccination failure is known to have occurred in ten dogs and four cats over 23 years.[120] An animal may fail to respond to vaccination if it is given too early (before three months of age in a kitten or puppy), if the animal's immune system is not functioning fully (immunocompromised) or if the animal is already incubating rabies.

However, the success of vaccination can be predicted by the use of serological testing, which involves testing the animal's blood for levels of antibody to rabies virus. Tests such as the rapid fluorescent focus inhibition test (RFFIT) are said to be accurate but require further work to ensure consistent results. RFFIT requires large scale processing for accurate results, facilities which are not available in all rabies-free and EU nations, including the UK. A reference serum, against which all tests could be measured, has yet to be agreed internationally. In addition, because of possible errors in serological testing, two such tests should be made.

Identification

Many of the potential problems arising from a system of vaccination are practical, rather than scientific. Is the animal entering Britain the same one identified on the vaccination certificate? Were the vaccination details recorded accurately? Could they have been forged? Unlike quarantine, where an animal can be observed in isolation for six months, a degree of trust is involved in vaccination procedures, whether this involves livestock, traded animals under the Balai Directive, or the recommendations of the Commons Select Committee on Agriculture, were they ever to be implemented. Under the former two systems, inspection is carried out in the country of origin and the importing country is notified in advance of the animal's arrival via the ANIMO computer system. There are no routine veterinary checks at the point of entry, but checks may be made at the final destination in the UK. Spot checks at borders may be carried out under certain circumstances. Thus such a system is more open to forgery or inadequate standards of certification. On health grounds, the information provided by the exporting country should be open to inspection at the border before the animal is allowed into Britain. Where doubt arises, confirmatory testing could be carried out.

   The most reliable way of identifying a dog or cat is by implanting it with a microchip. The chip may carry a unique identifying number which, for import purposes, gives access to the animal's health certification, which is carried on the ANIMO computer system and stored by MAFF. This would prevent the exchange of one animal for another. At present, however animals' microchip identification numbers are not included in the ANIMO system's data. Were an outbreak of rabies to occur, identification information would be useful in tracing these animals, particularly if they had since moved to another country.

   With these safeguards, fraudulent practice would still be possible, for instance by owners arranging for the replacement of another animal's blood samples for tests or the recording of incorrect information on the microchip. As the consequence of an animal's failing its serological testing could be six months of expensive quarantine, there may be considerable incentive for forgery. Also possible is the unintentional, but equally hazardous, recording of inaccurate information. However, when there is little to prevent smuggling within the European Union, it seems more feasible that an owner would attempt to bring the animal into the UK covertly rather than go to the trouble of forging or tampering with vaccination records.

Smuggling

Many argue that the expense and separation from a beloved pet caused by quarantine provide significant motives for animal smuggling and that the cheaper system of vaccination, where there is no period of isolation, would reduce this.[61] However, facts supporting this view are notably absent. Anecdotal evidence suggests that the smuggling of pets through seaports is relatively easy and it could equally be argued that any individual sufficiently irresponsible to risk introducing rabies into Britain is unlikely to go to the not inconsiderable trouble of following the vaccination procedures.

The system recommended by the Commons Select Committee on Agriculture would involve the pet having spent at least six months continuously in an approved country immediately before coming to the UK, being tattooed or implanted with a microchip, blood-tested four months after the vaccination and possibly given an annual booster vaccination. Following this an import licence would have to be obtained from MAFF specifying the point and time of entry into the UK and finally the Divisional Veterinary Officer responsible for the ultimate point of destination, who could subject the pet to a spot check, would also have to be informed. This process could cost around £70 to the owner and if the animal failed its serological test, it would still have to go into quarantine (costs estimated for 1995).

A risk assessment of Sweden's then proposed vaccination system, carried out by the Swedish Board of Agriculture, concluded 'It is by no means self-evident that smuggling will be reduced if the rules are altered' (from quarantine to vaccination and certification).[64] What is more, the replacement of quarantine with a system of vaccination has been interpreted by some as the relaxation or even abolition of Britain's rabies defences.[62,63] If such a perception is widely held, the threat posed by rabies may be underestimated and animal smuggling may actually increase. A public education campaign similar to that currently run by MAFF would be necessary to counteract such misconceptions.

Were rabies to enter Britain, the most likely vector would be a smuggled animal. It is therefore important that the risk is recognized and measures taken to prevent this illegal traffic before it is too late. Fines for those caught are at present about the same or less than the cost of putting a pet dog or cat in quarantine. Unless these penalties are substantially increased, smuggling will remain a risk worth taking.

Within EU law, border checks remain legal for Britain to protect itself from rabies on the grounds of protecting public health. However, if physical searches become less frequent due to fewer customs officers, alternative means of detecting smuggled animals must be found to detect hidden animals. In addition, the movement of traffic passing legally but rarely inspected into Britain from other EU nations remains a serious cause for concern.

Financial considerations of different policies

Vaccination and quarantine

Were the system of vaccination to prove as safe as quarantine, then the cost of importing and exporting pets would be spread more thinly among owners. More pets would be likely to travel but the cost to individual owners would be substantially lower than the fees for quarantine, costing between £70 and £130 (including serological testing and microchip identification) per animal, depending on the number of vaccinations and tests required, compared with around £1000 for a cat and £1200 for a dog in quarantine or the not inconsiderable expense of housing a pet in a commercial cattery or kennel in the owner's absence (costs estimated for 1995).

Essential to the viability of a vaccination, identification and serological testing scheme, would be the existence of a UK national reference laboratory for serological testing. International agreement is urgently needed on criteria for test standardization. Confirmatory serological testing of animals entering Britain would provide a further safeguard where there was doubt regarding the accuracy of animal health records.

It is estimated that there would be a substantial increase in dogs and cats travelling into Britain each year under a new scheme of vaccination and certification. If tests were required for all animals on entry, many animals would require one or possibly two tests in Britain. Even if only native British pets were required to be tested in this country (with imported EU pets being tested in the country of export), with increased ease of travel with the rest of Europe, the numbers are still likely to be very high. As no such facility is yet available in the UK, establishing one would demand considerable capital expenditure. Britain's current system of quarantine costs approximately £0.75 million to administer annually, including research projects.[70]

Chapter 10

Recommendations: strategies for prevention and control

The choices for keeping rabies out of Britain are retaining our current system of quarantine or introducing a system of vaccination in which the animal is serologically tested, certified and given a means of identification. As an option based on vaccination, certification and identification, the system recommended by the Commons Select Committee on Agriculture for Britain, is considered.

Two models for safeguarding Britain's future rabies-free status

The current system of quarantine

Quarantine regulations require six months quarantine for all dogs, cats, rabbits, mice, rats, gerbils, and most other rabies susceptible mammals except for dogs and cats included in the legislation following the Balai Directive (The Rabies (Importation of Dogs, Cats and Mammals) (Amendment) Order 1994), with anti-rabies vaccination of dogs and cats on entry under the Rabies (Importation of Dogs, Cats and Other Mammals) Order 1974 (as amended).

During transit to Britain the animal must be contained in a nose and paw proof container or crate, and in aircraft must travel as cargo in the freight compartment.

The animal may only be landed in Britain if:

• it has previously been issued with a British import licence

• arrangements have been made for the animal to undergo six months' quarantine in an approved quarantine kennel.

The animal may only be landed at certain specified ports or airports; it is an offence to land animals at any other port/airport unless in an emergency, and the animal will only be allowed to disembark with the permission of the local authority health inspector.

The animal must then be taken from the port of entry to quarantine premises by an authorized carrying agent.

The animal must be detained in quarantine for six months at the owner's expense. Quarantine may be extended in the case of a rabies outbreak at the quarantine premises.

Dogs and cats in quarantine must be vaccinated against rabies by the Veterinary Superintendent in charge as soon as practicable (with the exception of where it has been imported for research purposes with which vaccination might interfere).

Any animal in relation to which there are contraventions of or failure to comply with these requirements may be seized and, if appropriate, destroyed.

Animals from Northern Ireland, the Channel Islands, the Republic of Ireland or the Isle of Man do not have to fulfil these requirements unless they have been brought to those countries from elsewhere and have not undergone at least six months' quarantine before being landed in Britain.

The system proposed for dogs and cats by the Commons Select Committee on Agriculture

The following constitute the recommendations of the Commons Select Committee on Agriculture and were intended for immediate introduction:

- six months' quarantine should remain a requirement for all dogs and cats arriving from non-approved countries ('approved countries' being defined by the Commons Select Committee on Agriculture as 'internationally recognised to be rabies-free and carrying out appropriate policies to maintain their rabies-free status')

- dogs and cats intended to be imported into the UK from approved countries should:

  - be marked either by microchip or tattooed with a unique identifying number

- have spent at least six months continuously in an approved country immediately before becoming eligible to move on to the UK

- be vaccinated with an approved inactivated rabies vaccine at the age of three months or older

- four months after vaccination be blood-tested in an approved laboratory to determine whether there has been an adequate antibody response indicating that the animal is immune from rabies

• assuming the blood-test demonstrated the required level of protective antibodies, the animal would be permitted to enter the UK up to 12 months after the initial vaccination; if the animal travelled frequently between the UK and approved countries annual booster vaccinations would be necessary, though the animal could travel only one month after vaccination on the second and subsequent occasions, subject to a satisfactory blood-test

• prior to importation the owner would have to obtain an import licence from MAFF specifying port and time of entry into the UK; the Divisional Veterinary Officer responsible for the ultimate point of destination would also have to be informed. An animal's certification should be checked at the port of entry into the UK, and Divisional Veterinary Officers should carry out spot-checks at points of destination

• an animal's vaccination record and other health certification should be contained in a passport relating to the animal

• any infringement of these regulations would result at the very least in the animal's being quarantined or re-exported at the owner's expense, without prejudice to any further legal sanctions that might need to be taken

• quarantine would still be available for owners if an animal had failed blood-tests.[61]

Comment on these proposals

The Government has recently rejected the recommendations of the Commons Select Committee on Agriculture.[121] The BMA also considers that the recommendations of the Select Committee should not be implemented at present because there are insufficient safeguards to remove the risk of rabies entering Britain. The BMA's concerns include the following:

• using the boundary of the EU as Britain's outside boundary rather than the national boundary multiplies the points at which the system may fail:

- if the border controls of any member state of the EU are weak, an animal registered as resident in the EU may travel into and out of the Union unobserved, able to contract rabies in a non-EU country and return, without record of its movements

- evidence of weak links in the procedures necessary to prevent disease within the EU have already come to light with the reintroduction of warble fly to Britain since Britain lost responsibility for health inspection before entry

• widening the borders to include 'approved' rabies-free countries around the world would create further difficulties: the recommendations of the Commons Select Committee on Agriculture do not clarify how a country would be declared 'approved' as rabies free. Certain developing countries have reported no rabies cases, but doubts remain whether thorough surveillance can be assured. Rabies may reinfect a country and go unreported. There is at present no internationally accepted list of rabies-free countries

• reliance on the exporting countries (either EU or 'approved' rabies-free countries) for animals' health standards assumes:

- the availability of reliable facilities for serological testing of equal accuracy in all EU and 'approved' rabies-free countries

- equally high standards of training, competence and professional integrity for veterinary surgeons in EU and 'approved' rabies-free countries responsible for vaccination of animals, fitting of identification and accurate certification

- equally high standards of rabies surveillance in all 'approved' rabies-free countries

• tattoos are potentially unreliable, they may be 'doctored' easily and in some cases are difficult to inscribe legibly. Microchip implants should be fitted carrying the animal's identification thus allowing access to its health records.

The BMA's recommendations

The present system of quarantine with vaccination on entry should remain in place for dogs and cats (other than those covered by the Balai Directive) unless and until the following requirements can be fulfilled **in addition** to the system of vaccination, certification and identification recommended by the Commons Select Committee on Agriculture. These requirements would apply to cats and dogs from **current** EU member states and 'approved' rabies-free countries. These requirements would have to be the subject of special examination were additional members to join the EU.

Eligibility of countries

1   The Ministry of Agriculture, Fisheries and Food, as Britain's regulatory body for the import of live animals, should define those countries as 'approved' which it is satisfied fulfil the criteria set out by the Office International des Epizooties (OIE) as 'rabies-free' (see page 33).

2   Cats and dogs entering Britain from the EU should have spent a minimum of six months continuously in an EU member state before becoming eligible to enter Britain under a scheme of vaccination and certification.

Additional checks

3   Where point-of-entry checks give rise to insufficient confidence in the information supplied by the exporting nation, the right should be reserved for confirmatory antibody tests to be carried out in Britain on animals while awaiting leave to enter the country.

Additional safeguards for cats

4   Research evidence regarding the efficacy of vaccines remains less comprehensive for cats than dogs. Stricter requirements for cats should therefore be considered.

Serological testing

5   A fully equipped national reference laboratory capable of carrying out large numbers of the RFFIT or acceptable alternatives for serological testing should be set up in the UK. Similar facilities would be required in all countries exporting cats and dogs to Britain. Criteria for test standardization and appropriate internal and external quality control must be established and agreed internationally.

6   At an appropriate interval following vaccination, two serological tests (both using RFFIT or an acceptable alternative) should be carried out at an approved laboratory on sera collected separately (the WHO recommend that the two sera samples be collected at least 4 weeks apart) in the exporting country.[111] The results of the two tests must be positive for the required antibody level.

7   Importation of animals into Britain should be restricted to those ports with the facilities for holding animals when additional serological testing is considered necessary.

Identification and documentation

8   A European standard should be agreed for microchip identification implants and their readers ensuring compatibility throughout the European Union.

9   The ANIMO (ANImal MOvements) computer-based information system, currently used for livestock and cats and dogs entering Britain under the Balai Directive, should be used to enable the rapid transfer of information regarding other cats and dogs moving between countries and into Britain.

10 In order to trace the movement of imported animals in the case of an actual or suspected outbreak of rabies, the European Commission should require that the microchip implant identification details be recorded on the ANIMO system in addition to other details and retained in long-term records.

Further requirements

11 For animals entering the EU from rabies endemic areas, countries in the EU must agree minimum standards of inspection, rabies vaccination, identification, and documentation.

Legislation

12 Legislation should be enacted to ensure that all these measures (1 to 12 above) can be successfully achieved before there is any change from the current system of quarantine to a system of vaccination, certification and identification.

In the absence of such legislation the BMA recommends that the current quarantine requirements be retained for cats and dogs.

Additional recommendations

Advice to travellers

13 GPs and travel agents should be provided with up-to-date information to advise those travelling to rabies enzootic countries of the precautions to be taken and actions needed following suspected exposure to the virus.

Smuggling

14 Higher penalties are needed to deter smuggling of unprotected animals. These should include higher fines and possible imprisonment together with the option of destroying the animal.

15 Surveillance techniques which could detect animals left in vehicles or luggage, should be employed at all British ports and airports with wide advertisement of the presence of such devices.

Research

16 Research into methods of rabies control should continue to be encouraged and funded, including means of vaccinating wildlife in urban areas; the most efficient, economical ways of immunizing humans and domestic animals should be investigated.

Vaccines

17 The French purified vero cell vaccine and the German purified chick embryo cell vaccine should be licensed for use in Britain as a money-saving measure.

Rabies vaccines ancient and modern for human use

Vaccines prepared from nervous tissue

Many, although not all, of the strains of fixed virus used for vaccine production throughout the world are derivatives of the 'Pasteur' virus isolated and maintained in Paris for more than a century. The deaths occurring among those undergoing treatment, although statistically small, were seized upon by Pasteur's critics. They remarked upon the hazards of inoculating crude material which almost certainly contained live, albeit attenuated virus. *Rage du laboratoire* (laboratory acquired rabies) was hence sometimes unkindly called 'Pasteur's disease', perhaps the most valid of the criticisms of Pasteur's techniques of the time. The 'Pasteur' method remained the treatment of choice in France and her colonies for more than 50 years.

Modifications to the vaccine soon began to be introduced in the early 1900s, spinal cords were replaced by whole brain and methods were directed toward partial or complete inactivation of the virus by heat or chemicals. Notable among these modifications was that of Semple, an Englishman working in India, who in 1911 prepared vaccine in which virus was killed by incubating suspensions of infected brain with phenol. Despite the allergic encephalomyelitic reactions which occur with vaccine produced in adult mammalian brain, Semple-type vaccine became the most widely used of the rabies vaccines. Although far superior vaccines are now available, in many parts of the developing world, Semple vaccine is still used, notably in India, largely because it is the cheapest vaccine and the infected neural tissues of adult mammals – rabbits, sheep, goats – provide abundant sources of virus for vaccine production; ß-propiolactone has replaced phenol as an inactivant.

The unmyelinated central nervous system (CNS) of newborn mammals is relatively free from neuroallergen and rabies virus multiplies to high titre in the brains of immature animals. An inactivated vaccine prepared in suckling mouse brain (SMB) is of high potency and remains the favoured product in Latin America.

The incidence of neurological side effects with this vaccine is reputedly a quarter to a fifth that of Semple-type vaccine. Current recommendations suggest that if mice no older than one day are used and brain suspensions are centrifuged, neuroallergens are further reduced in the final product. SMB vaccine is used in humans but is also widely used for immunizing dogs, cats and cattle. It has been administered to many millions of dogs since its initial field trials in 1960.

Vaccines prepared in avian embryos

Avian embryos began to be used for growing viruses during the Second World War. Duck embryo vaccine (DEV) was developed during the same period. Because of its virtual freedom from neuroallergens it was adopted as a much safer vaccine for human use; in the USA and Britain it replaced nervous tissue vaccines until the advent of products produced in cell cultures. Many believed that its immunogenicity was poor and that potency was sacrificed for safety. None of these strictures apply to the modern purified and highly potent DEV now produced in Switzerland.

Vaccines produced in cell cultures

What has been described as a second generation of safer and more potent rabies vaccines began to appear after the serial propagation of the virus in cultures of non-neural cells by Kissling (1958). The virus harvested from suitable cell cultures was more readily purified than material from brain suspensions and information on virus structure, biophysical and antigenic properties became available. Although rabies is a highly neurotropic virus (i.e. it has a marked affinity for nerve cells), after a period of adaptation, it will grow *in vitro* in a wide variety of mammalian and avian cells. Rabies vaccines currently available for human use are summarized in Tables 9 and 10.

These notes illuminate some of the achievements, problems and direction that has accompanied rabies vaccine development over the past century. The introduction of any new vaccine requires the approval of the national licensing authority and it must satisfy the basic requirements of any vaccine. Evidence, indicative of efficacy, safety, stability, continuity of production and its ability to induce durable immunity is fundamental.

Table 9 Inactivated tissue culture rabies vaccines for human use

Vaccine	Cell line	Virus strain	Country of origin	Date first licensed
Human diploid cell (HDCV)	human diploid cells	PM1503 PM1503 SAD CL-77	France Germany Canada	1974 1978 1985
Hamster kidney cell	primary hamster kidney cells	Vnukovo-32	USSR	1975
Dog kidney cell	primary dog kidney cells	PM 1503	Netherlands	1978
Chick embryo cell	primary chick embryo cells	HEP	Japan	1980
Hamster kidney cell	primary hamster kidney cells	Beijing-31	China	1981
Purified chick embryo cell (PCEC)	primary chick embryo cells	LEP	Germany	1985
Purified vero cell vaccine (PVRV)	African green monkey kidney cells	PM 1503	France	1985
Rabies vaccine absorbed (RVA)	Diploid fetal rhesus lung cell	Kissling	USA	1988
Purified duck embryo (PDEV)	Duck embryos (not a tissue culture vaccine)	PM	Switzerland	1985

Table 10 Summary of modern rabies vaccines for human use and treatment regimens in western Europe (and widely exported)

• human diploid cell vaccine (HDCV) (Imovax rabies, Pasteur-Mérieux) dose = 1 ml. The only vaccine currently available in the UK
• purified chick embryo cell vaccine (PCEC) (Rabipur, Behring) dose = 1 ml
• purified vero cell vaccine (PVRV) (Verorab, Pasteur-Mérieux) dose = 0.5 ml
• purified duck embryo vaccine (PDEV) (Lyssavac-N, Berna) dose = 1 ml. Not used with intradermal regimens

• post-exposure regimens
  – standard intramuscular (IM) regimen: five doses
    One dose IM into the deltoid on days 0, 3, 7, 14 and 30
 	
  – Economical multisite intradermal regimens have been developed for use in tropical endemic areas, but are also appropriate for Western use. There is a 60% reduction in the amount of vaccine used[122]

(post-exposure treatments also include wound care and giving rabies immunoglobulin)

• pre-exposure regimens
  – intramuscular regimen: three doses.
    One dose IM into the deltoid on days 0, 7 and 28
    A booster dose after one year is recommended
 	
  – intradermal (ID) regimen with HDCV, PVRV or PCEC
    0.1 ml of vaccine given ID at the same intervals

See detailed instructions for use elsewhere (CDC 1991, Rabies prevention – United States, (1991) *Morbid Mortal Wkly Rpt* 40 RR-3). *Immunisation against Infectious Diseases* (1992), HMSO London. New recommendations for intradermal vaccine regimens are to be published by WHO in 1995/1996

Vaccines for animals (including oral vaccination of foxes)

Vaccines prepared in avian embryos

A strain of virus named after its unfortunate victim 'Flury', isolated from human brain was established in chick embryos by Koprowski and Cox (1948). Vaccines are suspensions of embryo tissue containing living virus at different passage levels. Flury LEP (low egg passage) is antigenic in adult dogs although it retains some virulence for puppies, cats, cattle and some exotic species.

Flury HEP (high egg passage) is further attenuated and was licensed for cats and cattle. Trials in man were disappointing. The Flury virus strains adapted to cell-culture are still much used in vaccines. Some workers found they were more immunogenic in dogs than inactivated vaccines and gave more durable immunity after a single dose. Nevertheless, the use of live rabies vaccines is declining with the development of more inactivated products with high potency.

Oral vaccines for foxes

The possibility of controlling rabies in wildlife by immunization rather than by population reduction has been vigorously investigated for more than 30 years. Four types of oral live virus vaccines have been developed for distribution to the dominant vector species in Europe, the red fox (*Vulpes vulpes*). Attenuated rabies viruses were introduced first, followed by a genetically engineered vaccinia recombinant virus.

Attenuated live rabies vaccines

Inactivated vaccines are not immunogenic when given orally and for this reason oral vaccines have used attenuated viruses.[123] Those used in the live oral vaccines are derivatives of the fixed SAD (Street Alabama Dufferin) strain, originally from a dog in Alabama.

The Bern strain of SAD virus was immunogenic and harmless when given orally to foxes. Although it was thoroughly tested for pathogenicity in non-target species, there is some evidence that this lack of infectivity (avirulence) might not be a stable characteristic. The vaccine initially used for fox vaccination in Europe has killed baboons and also, in certain circumstances, laboratory rodents, although there is no evidence that it can establish an infectious cycle in the latter.[124]

Another derivative of the SAD strain, SAD B19, was also used in the field, but concern about reversion to virulence led to a further development. In 1990 SAG 1, a mutant of the SAD virus prepared in the laboratory and lacking a particular amino acid associated with virulence, was introduced in France.[125]

Recently SAG 2, an avirulent mutant double of the SAD Bern virus has been produced. Because two nucleotides are altered at position 333 on the glycoprotein gene, the chance of reversion to virulence is remote. The virus is immunogenic and stable, and field trials are awaited.[126]

Genetic recombinant vaccine

Glycoprotein is the basic component of the projections which cover the surface of rabies virus particles. The intact protein induces a strong immune response, inducing virus-neutralizing antibody which protects animals against lethal infection with rabies virus.[127] Rabies glycoprotein would be potentially useful as a vaccine, but large scale production has proved difficult. The use of rabies glycoprotein has been advanced by technological developments that enabled the construction of recombinant viruses. The gene coding for rabies virus glycoprotein is introduced into the genome of an attenuated vaccinia virus. The glycoprotein is expressed (produced) during viral replication. This recombinant vaccine (V-RG) proved safe when given orally to mice, rats, rabbits, cats, dogs, sheep, ferrets, badgers, hedgehogs and wild boar, and also subcutaneously to cattle.[128] A more recent recombinant using infectious human adenovirus for expressing rabies G-protein shows promise as a future oral vaccine for dogs in endemic areas.[129]

The WHO Expert Committee on Rabies, avers that over the past eight years V-RG 'was not pathogenic in over ten avian and 35 mammalian species'.[111] Since 1989 more than two million doses have been used in highly successful field trials in Belgium and France.[50]

Testing rabies vaccines

Whenever those concerned with the manufacture and control of rabies vaccines meet, discussion inevitably turns to the inadequacies of the currently accepted methods for assessing potency. The NIH test for potency was developed in the National Institutes of Health in the USA nearly 40 years ago.[130] Directly or indirectly it has been the subject of numerous international collaborative evaluations.

It is what the theorists call an antigen extinction test and involves the immunization of groups of mice with dilutions of test and reference vaccines followed by an intracerebral challenge with a standard strain of virus. It is criticized because its reproducibility is poor, it does not simulate the normal conditions of use of the vaccine, there is wide variability in results between different laboratories and more recent evidence suggests that differences between the virus used for producing the vaccine and the virus used for challenging the mice can further influence the results of potency assays.[131,132] No acceptable replacement has yet been found for the NIH test and it remains the subject of argument and review although alternative tests have been suggested.

A single radial immunodiffusion (SRD) test for estimating the glycoprotein content of vaccine as a measure of potency is well established, and an antibody induction test involving the assay of neutralizing antibody in mice immunized with dilutions of vaccine has been developed. Antibody binding and Enzyme linked immuno sorbent assay (ELISA) have also been developed as *in vitro* methods for estimating vaccine potency.[133]

Antibody is a fundamental element in the response to most vaccines and it was concluded that the NIH test in mice measured antibody immune response to vaccine.[134] There is evidence of a direct relationship between antibody titres and protection from challenge in dogs and cats.[107] The relative ease with which antibody can be measured has made it a convenient indicator of immune responses to vaccine.

There are many tests for estimating antibody to rabies virus: they include the classic serological techniques of complement fixation, passive and direct haemagglutination, reduction of viral plaques in cell-culture, radio immunoassay and a comparatively new passive agglutination test using latex beads sensitized with rabies antigen. Some of these methods were subjected to rigorous statistical assessment of the antibody titrations on the sera of 55 vaccinated dogs.[135] Many of these tests are seldom used and three methods are most commonly used.

Mouse neutralization test (MNT)

In the MNT test, serial dilutions of serum containing antibodies are mixed with a constant dose of standard challenge virus; the mixtures are incubated at 37° for 90 minutes for neutralization to occur, and then inoculated intracerebrally into suckling mice. A standard reference serum is titrated at the same time. Five mice are inoculated with each serum virus mixture and the number of mice dying between the sixth and 20th day after inoculation is recorded; the serum dilution at which 50% of the mice would survive can be calculated and antibody titres expressed as international units by reference to the standard. It is time consuming and it takes three weeks to obtain a result. All biological tests involving living animals should be avoided and results can be variable. It entails the use of live rabies virus, which in England necessitates special containment facilities. Mouse neutralization test (MNT) has proven less reliable than the rapid fluorescent focus inhibition test (RFFIT) in a study comparing the results of nine different laboratories.[109]

Rapid fluorescent focus inhibition test (RFFIT)

The RFFIT is similar in principle, but instead of mice being inoculated with serum + virus mixtures, cell cultures are inoculated. After 24 hours incubation the cells are examined by fluorescent antibody staining for the presence of non-neutralized virus. A specific number of microscope fields are examined for each serum dilution and the reduction of 50% in the number with fluorescent cells indicate the end point of neutralization. Results can be obtained within 48 hours instead of three weeks. The results tend to be lower than those determined in mice and discrepancies are reported, including difficulties of compatibility with the sera of dogs and the cell substrate used in the test. Immunofluorescence microscope facilities are needed and objectivity in assessing fluorescent cells may be difficult for those without considerable experience and technical ability. The same reservations concerning the handling of live rabies virus apply.*

*Both these methods are described in detail in *Laboratory Techniques in Rabies* 1973 (3rd edn.) (eds Kaplan MM and Koprowski H) WHO, Geneva. pp. 314 and 35.

Enzyme linked immuno sorbent assay (ELISA)

In ELISA, reactions of antibody with antigen take place with one or other component firmly attached to a solid base, in for example, the wells of multititre plates. Antigen or antibody is conjugated to an indicator enzyme (usually peroxidase) whose presence is detected by adding substrate that is converted to a coloured product by the action of the enzyme. The colour can be recorded visually or measured in a spectrophotometer and its intensity is proportional to the amount of labelled antigen or antibody bound in the test.

The advantages of the ELISA are said to be sensitivity, stability, safety, speed and economy. On the debit side non-specific binding occurs so that there are dangers of false positives.[136,137]

References

1   Pollard J (1964) *Wolves and Werewolves*. Robert Hale, London.

2   Committee of Inquiry on Rabies (1971) *Final Report*. HMSO, London.

3   Steele J H, Fernandez P J (1991) History of rabies and global aspects. In: *The natural history of rabies*. (2nd edn.) Baer G M, ed. CRC Press, Boca Raton, USA: 1–24.

4   Dunlop J M (1978) A hair of the dog. *J Roy Coll Gen Pract*. **28**: 293–6.

5   Bynum W F (1994) *Science and the practice of medicine in the nineteenth century*. Cambridge University Press, Cambridge.

6   Hill F J (1991) Keeping Britain free of rabies, *Proc R Soc Med* (1971). **64**: 213. Cited in Steel J H, Fernandez P J *History of rabies and global aspects*. In: *The natural history of rabies*. (2nd edn.) Baer G M, ed. CRC Press, Boca Raton, USA: 1–24.

7   Turner T (1984) The risks and problems associated with the importation of dogs, cats and other mammals: I Rabies. *Br Vet J*. **140**: 96–106.

8   Question of Rabies (1970) *New Scientist*, 19 March.

9   Botting J (1993) Rabies: a century of research brings eradication closer. *RDS News*, October: 8–12.

10   Pastoret P-P, Boulanger D, Brochien B. The rabies situation in Europe. *Veterinary Annual*, (in press).

11   Kaplan C, Turner G S, Warrell D A (1986) *Rabies: the facts*. 2nd edn. Oxford University Press, Oxford.

12   WHO Collaborating Centre for Rabies Surveillance and Research. (1994) *Rabies Bulletin* Europe **1/94: 18.**

13   Steele J H (1988) Rabies in the Americas and remarks on global aspects. *J Inf Dis* **10, Suppl 4:** 5585–97.

14   Bögel K, Motschwiller E (1986) Incidence of rabies and post–exposure treatment in developing countries. *Bulletin* WHO **64:** 883–7.

15   Familusi J B, Osunkoya B O, Moore D L *et al.* (1972) A fatal human infection with Mokola virus. *Am J Trop Med Hyg* **21:** 959–63.

16   Meridith C D, Rossouw A P, van Praag Koch H (1971) An unusual case of human rabies thought to be of chiropteran origin. *S Afr Med J* **45:** 767–9.

17   Adapted from King A A, Crick J (1988) *Rabies–related viruses.* In: Campbell J M, Charlton K M, eds. *Rabies.* Kluwer Academic Publishers, 177–99, London.

18   Department of Health and Social Security and the Welsh Office. (1977) *Memorandum on rabies.* London: HMSO.

19   Tillotson J R, Axelrod D, Lyman D O (1977) *MMWR* **26:** 249–50.

20   Warrell D A, Davidson N McD, Pope H M, *et al.* (1976) Pathophysiological studies in human rabies, *Am J Med* **60:** 180–90.

21   Human rabies – California. (1994) *JAMA* **272:** 347–9.

22   Originally published in Kaplan C, Turner G S and Warrell D A (1986) *Rabies: the Facts.* 2nd edn. Oxford University Press, Oxford: 43–5.

23   Walker E, Williams G, Raeside F. eds. (1993) *ABC of healthy travel.* BMJ, London.

24   Ministry of Agriculture, Fisheries and Food (1994) *Rabies prevention and control.* MAFF publications, London.

25   *The Rabies (Importation of Dogs, Cats and Mammals) (Amendment) Order,* (1994) HMSO, London.

26   Thiriart C, Ioken A, Costy F, *et al.* (1985) Immunization of young foxes against rabies: interaction between vaccination and natural infection. *Annales de Recherches Veterinarires,* **16:** 289–92.

27   WHO Information System (1994) *Summary for the WHO European Region.* WHO/EPI/CEIS/94.2 EU, August.

28   Blancou J (1988) *Epizootiology of rabies: Eurasia and Africa.* In: Campbell J M, Charlton K M, eds. *Rabies.* Kluwer Academic Publishers, London: 243–65.

29   Meslin F-X, Fishbein D B, Matter H C (1994) Rationale and prospects for rabies elimination in developing countries. *Current topics in Microbiology and Immunology.* **187** *Lyssaviruses:* 1–26.

30   Petricciani J C (1993) Ongoing tragedy of rabies. *Lancet* **342:** 1067.

31   Lum C W S (1994) Maintenance of rabies-free status and quarantine requirements for the state of Hawaii, In: *Report of the expert consultation on the technical bases for recognition of rabies-free areas and animal quarantine requirements,* 21–2 November, Santo Domingo, Dominican Republic, (In press).

32   Doyle K (1994) Maintenance of rabies-free status and quarantine requirements – Australia, In: *Report of the expert consultation on the technical bases for recognition of rabies-free areas and animal quarantine requirements,* 21–2 November, Santo Domingo, Dominican Republic, (In press).

33   O'Neil B (1994) Maintenance of New Zealand's rabies-free status and quarantine requirements, In: *Report of the expert consultation on the technical bases for recognition of rabies-free areas and animal quarantine requirements,* 21–2 November, Santo Domingo, Dominican Republic, (In press).

34   World Health Organization (1990) *Report of a WHO/NVI workshop on Arctic rabies.* Uppsala, Sweden, 24–7 April 1990. WHO, Geneva.

35   Baer G M (1991) Vampire bat and bovine paralytic rabies. In: *The natural history of rabies.* Baer G M, ed. 2nd edn. CRC Press, Boca Raton, USA: 389–403.

36   Lumio J, Hillbom M, Roine R, *et al.* (1986) Human rabies of bat origin in Europe. *Lancet;* **i:** 378.

37   Follman E H, Ritter D G, Beller M (1994) Survey of fox trappers in northern Alaska for rabies antibody. *Epidmiol Infec.* **113:** 137–41.

38   WHO Rabies Res. 93.39 (1993) *Report of the first seminar on the control of rabies in English speaking West African countries.* Geneva: WHO.

39   Smith J S, Baer G M (1988) *Epizootiology of rabies: the Americas.* In: Campbell J M, Charlton K M, eds. *Rabies.* Kluwer Academic Publishers, London: 267–99.

40   Spencer L M (1994) Taking the bite out of rabies, report of meeting 'Advances towards rabies control in the Americas'. Philadelphia, October 1993. *J Am Vet Med Ass.* **204:** 479–84.

41   Everard C O R, Everard J D (1992) Mongoose rabies in the Caribbean. *Annals of the New York Academy of Sciences.* **653:** 356–66.

42   Agriculture Committee (1994) *Fifth Report. Health controls on the importation of live animals.* Volume II. HMSO, London.

43   Articles 30 to 36 of the Treaty of Rome, as amended by the Single European Act.

44   Article 36 and paragraphs 3 and 4 of Article 100A of the Treaty of Rome, as amended by the Single European Act.

45   Officer van Juslite v De Peiper, Case 104/75 (1976) ECR 613, (1976) 2 CMLR 271, para 16. (1992) In: Fine F L. 'Foodstuffs with additives: free movement within the EC'. *British Food J.* **94, No 8:** 30.

46   Van Bebbejin (1983) ECR. Cited in Weathergill S. Food scares and the Treaty of Rome. (1989) *The Law Society Gazette* **14:** 15.

47   Wilhelm U, Schneider L G (1990) Oral immunization of foxes against rabies: practical experiences of a field trial in the Federal Republic of Germany. *Bulletin of the World Health Organization.* **68:** 87–92.

48   Wandeler A, Steck F, Bichel P, Capt S, Schneider L (1982) Oral immunisation of foxes against rabies – a field study. *ABL Vet Med B.* **29:** 372–96.

49   Wandeler A I (1988) *Control of rabies in wildlife.* In: Campbell J M, Charlton K M, eds. *Rabies.* Kluwer Academic Publishers, London: 365–80.

50   Sureau P (1992) Contribution to rabies prevention. *Vaccine.* **10:** 896–9.

51   WHO Collaborating Centre for Rabies Surveillance and Research. (1993) *Rabies Bulletin Europe.* **4/92:** 16.

52   Aubert M, Masson E, Vuillaume P, Artois M, Barrat J (1993) Les acquis de la prophylaxie contre la rage vulpine en France. *Méd Mal Infect,* **23** Spéciale: 537–45.

53   MacKenzie D (1994) Europe launches spring offensive against rabies. *New Scientist,* 30 April. 6–7.

54   Jackson C (1993) Hopes for an EC free of rabies. *The Times,* 8 July.

55   King A, Davies P (1988) Bat rabies. *State Vet J.* **42:** 140–8.

56   Petkevicius S (1993) Oral vaccination of wild animals against rabies as practised in Lithuania. WHO Collaborating Centre for Rabies Surveillance and Research, *Rabies Bulletin Europe 1/93.* **17:** 10–11.

57   WHO Collaborating Centre for Rabies Surveillance and Research (1991) *Rabies Bulletin Europe 3/91.* **15.**

58   Steck F, Wandeler A I. The epidemiology of fox rabies in Europe. *Epidemiologic Reviews 1980;* **2:** 71–96, cited in Pastoret P-P, *The rabies situation in Europe.* Veterinary Annual (In press).

59   Artois M, Aubert M F A (1985) *Behaviour of rabid foxes.* In: Artois M, Blancou J, Kempf C, eds. Ecology and epidemiology of wild and feral canids in the Paleartic zone. *Revue d'Ecologie (la Terre et la Vie).* **40:** 171–6, cited in Pastoret P-P, *The rabies situation in Europe.* Veterinary Annual (In press).

60   Memorandum by the Association of Port Health Authorities Agriculture Committee, Appendix 30. Fifth Report (1994) *Health controls on the importation of live animals.* Volume II. HMSO, London.

61   Agriculture Committee (1994) Fifth Report. *Health controls on the importation of live animals.* Volume I. HMSO, London.

62   Quarantine rules change as rabies defences weaken (1994) *The Independent,* 15 January.

63   'Britain should drop control on rabies' say MPs (1994) *Daily Telegraph,* 23 November.

64   Swedish Board of Agriculture (1992) *Considerations concerning import regulations governing dogs and cats with regard to the risks of the introduction of rabies.* Memorandum from the Infection Protection Unit, (unpublished).

65   Aubert M (1994) Control of rabies in foxes: what are the appropriate measures? *Veterinary Record.* **134:** 55–9.

66   Harris S, Rayner J M V (1986) A discriminant analysis of the current distribution of urban foxes *(Vulpes vulpes)* in Britain. *J of Animal Ecology.* **55:** 605–11.

67   Trewhella W J, Harris S, McAllister F E (1988) Dispersal distance, home-range size and population density in the red fox (*Vulpes vulpes*): a quantitative analysis. *J of Applied Ecology.* **25:** 423–34.

68   Harris S, Smith G C (1987) The use of sociological data to explain the distribution and numbers of urban foxes *(Vulpes vulpes)* in England and Wales. *Symposia of the Zoological Society of London.* **58:** 313–28.

69   Office of Population Censuses and Surveys (1984) *Census 1981: Key Statistics for Urban Areas: Great Britain.* HMSO, London.

70   King A A, Turner G S (1993) Rabies: a review. *J of Comparative Pathology.* **108:** 1–39.

71   Blancou J (1988) Ecology and epidemiology of fox rabies. *Rev Inf Dis.* **10 Suppl 4:** S606–S609.

72   Stebbings R E (1991) *Order chiroptera – introduction.* In: Corbet
     G B, Harris S, eds. *The handbook of British mammals.* 3rd edn.
     Blackwell Scientific Publications, Oxford. 81–6.

73   Hutson A M (1991) *Serotine Eptesicus serotinus* In: Corbet G B,
     Harris S, eds. *The handbook of British mammals.* 3rd edn.
     Blackwell Scientific Publications, Oxford. 112–16.

74   Juedes U (1987) Zum problem der Tollwut bei Fledermausen.
     Myotis. **25:** 41–59.

75   Trewhella W J, Harris S, Smith G C, Nadian A K (1991) A field
     trial evaluating bait uptake by an urban fox *(Vulpes vulpes)*
     population. *J of Applied Ecology.* **28:** 454–66.

76   Wandeler A I, Capt S, Gerber H, Kappeler A, Kipfer R (1988)
     Rabies epidemiology, natural barriers and fox vaccination.
     Parassitologia. **30:** 53–7.

77   Harris S, Cheeseman C L, Smith G C, Trewhella W J (1992) Rabies
     contingency planning in Britain. In: O'Brien P, Berry G, eds.
     Wildlife rabies: contingency planning in Australia. Proceedings No.
     11, Canberra: AGPS Bureau of Rural Resources, 63–77.

78   The Pet Food Manufacturers Association (1995) *Profile 1995.* The
     Pet Food Manufacturers Association, London.

79   Nicholson G (1981) *Government policy on rabies control.* In: *The
     ecology and control of feral cats.* Potters Bar: UFAW, 50–9.

80   Harris S, Morris P, Wray S, Yalden D (1994) *A review of British
     mammals – population estimates and conservation status of British
     mammals other than cetaceans.* Joint Nature Conservation
     Committee, Peterborough.

81   Rees P (1981) The ecological distribution of feral cats and the
     effects of neutering a hospital colony. In: *The ecology and control
     of feral cats.* Potters Bar: UFAW, 12–22.

82   Harris S, Rayner J M V (1986) Models for predicting urban fox
     (*Vulpes vulpes*) numbers in British cities and their application for
     rabies control. *J of Animal Ecology.* **55:** 593–603.

83   Saunders G, White P C L, Harris S, Rayner J M V (1993) Urban foxes: food acquisition, time and energy budgeting of a generalised predator. *Symposia of the Zoological Society of London.* **65:** 215–34.

84   Harris S, Smith G C (1987) Demography of two urban fox (*Vulpes vulpes*) populations. *J of Applied Ecology.* **24:** 75–86.

85   Harris S, Trewhella W J (1988) An analysis of some of the factors affecting dispersal in an urban fox (*Vulpes vulpes*) population. *J of Applied Ecology.* **25:** 409–22.

86   Smith G C, Harris S (1991) Rabies in urban foxes (*Vulpes vulpes*) in Britain: the use of a spatial stochastic simulation model to examine the pattern of spread and evaluate the efficacy of different control régimes. *Philosophical Transactions of the Royal Society of London.* **334:** 459–79.

87   White P C L, Harris S (1994) Encounters between red foxes (*Vulpes vulpes*): implications for territory maintenance, social cohesion and dispersal. *J of Animal Ecology.* **63:** 315–27.

88   White P C L, Harris S, Smith G C (1995) Fox contact behaviour and rabies spread: a model for the estimation of contact probabilities between urban foxes at different population densities and its implications for rabies control in Britain. *J of Applied Ecology.* (In press).

89   WHO Collaborating Centre for Rabies Surveillance and Research. (1993) *Rabies Bulletin Europe.* **1/93:** 17.

90   Cresswell W J, Harris S, Bunce R G H, Jefferies D J (1989) The badger (*Meles meles*) in Britain: present status and future population changes. *Biological J of the Linnean Society.* **38:** 91–101.

91   Downing G (1990) Mad dogs and fieldsportsmen. *Shooting Times & Country Magazine.* **4596:** 15.

92   Adapted from Cresswell W J, Harris S, Jefferies D J (1990) *The history, distribution, status and habitat requirements of the badger in Britain.* Nature Conservancy Council, Peterborough.

93   Anderson R M, Jackson H C, May R M, Smith A D M (1981)
     Population dynamics of fox rabies in Europe. *Nature,* 26 February.
     289: 765–71.

94   WHO Collaborating Centre for Rabies Surveillance and Research
     (1993) *Rabies Bulletin Europe.* **4/92:** 16.

95   Department of Trade and Industry Consumer Safety Unit (1992)
     Home and leisure accident research (1992 data). Department of
     Trade and Industry, London.

96   British Medical Association (1990) *The BMA guide to living with
     risk.* Penguin, Harmondsworth.

97   Cheeseman C L, Wilesmith J W, Ryan J, Mallinson P J (1987)
     Badger population dynamics in a high-density area. *Symposia of
     the Zoological Society of London.* **58:** 279–94.

98   Velander K A (1991) Pine marten *Martes martes* In: Corbet G B,
     Harris S, eds. *The handbook of British mammals.* 3rd edn.
     Blackwell Scientific Publications, Oxford. 368–76.

99   Directorate–General for Agriculture (1992) *Report of a sub-group
     of the Scientific Veterinary Committee on various aspects of rabies.*
     Commission of the European Communities. (unpublished).

100 King A (1992) *Current application of quarantine measures world
     wide – new trends.* OIE Rabies Control, April. 15–18.

101 Gawler J S H (1994) *Investigation into the necessity of Britain's six
     months quarantine period for domestic cats and dogs.* BA
     dissertation, (unpublished).

102 Blancou J, Aubert M F A, Soulebot J P (1963) Differences dans le
     pouvoir pathogene de souches de virus rabique adapts au renard au
     chien. *Ann Virol.* **134E:** 523–31.

103 Klintevall K (1994) Rabies vaccination and antibody testing in lieu
     of dog quarantine in Sweden. In: *Report of the expert consultation
     on the technical bases for recognition of rabies-free areas and
     animal quarantine requirements,* 21–2 November, Santo Domingo,
     Dominican Republic, (In press).

104   Bakken G (1994) *Rabies vaccination and antibody testing in lieu of quarantine – New requirements for dogs and cats imported to Norway and Sweden from European countries of the EU/EFTA*, In: *Report of the expert consultation on the technical bases for recognition of rabies-free areas and animal quarantine requirements*, 21–2 November, Santo Domingo, Dominican Republic, (In press).

105   Aubert M F A (1992) *Results of a survey on rabies vaccination and quarantine for domestic carnivora in western Europe*, OIE Rabies Control, April. 1–7.

106   Aubert M F A (1992) Practical significance of rabies antibody in cats and dogs. *Revue Scientifique et Technique Off Int Epiz.* **11**: 735–60.

107   Aubert M F A (1993) Can vaccination validated by the titration of rabies antibodies in serum of cats and dogs be an alternative to quarantine measures? *Abstracts on hygiene and communicable diseases.* **68**: R1–R21.

108   Smith J S, Yager P A, Baer G M (1973) A rapid reproducible test for determining neutralizing antibody. *Bull WHO.* **48**: 535–41.

109   Lyng J (1994) Calibration of a replacement preparation for the international standard for rabies immunoglobulin. *Biologicals.* **22**: 249–55.

110   Aubert M F A (1994) Personal communication with A King.

111   WHO Expert Committee on Rabies (1992) *Eighth report.* WHO technical report series, 824. Geneva: World Health Organization.

112   (1994) Commission Decision 18th April 1994 laying down system of ID for dogs/cats placed on the market in UK from EU Countries, 94/274/EC. *Official Journal of the European Communities.* 7 May, No L 117/40.

113   Fontaine R E, Schantz P M. Pet ownership and knowledge of zoonotic diseases in DC Kalb County, Georgia. *Anthrozoos.* **III**: 45–9.

114   Cundy J M (1980) Rabies encephalitis: management in a district general hospital ICU. *Anaesthesia.* **35**: 35–41.

115   Meredith C (1994) MAFF, Personal communication with S Mars.

116   Sudarskis A (1994) Rhône Mérieux, Personal communication with S Mars.

117   (1992) *Calculations derived from those in Swedish Board of Agriculture. Considerations concerning import regulations governing dogs and cats with regard to the risks of the introduction of rabies.* Memorandum from the Infection Protection Unit, (unpublished).

118   WHO Collaborating Centre for Rabies Surveillance and Research (1994) *Rabies Bulletin Europe.* **2/94:** 18.

119   Fishbein D B (1991) Rabies in humans. In: *The natural history of rabies.* Baer G M, ed. 2nd edn. CRC Press, Boca Raton, USA: 519–51.

120   Aubert M F A, Barrat J. (1992) Les échecs de vaccinations chez les animaux domestiques. *Bull Epidémiol mensuel Rage anim France* 1991; 21: 1. In: Aubert M F A. Practical significance of rabies antibodies in cats and dogs. *Revue Scientifique et Technique Off Int Epiz.* **11:** 735–60.

121   Ministry of Agriculture, Fisheries and Food (1995) *The Government reply to the fifth report from the Agriculture Committee Session 1993–94. Health Controls on the Import of Live Animals.* HMSO, London.

122   Warrell M J, Nicholson K N, Warrell D A *et al.* (1985) Economical multiple–site intradermal immunisation with human diploid-cell strain vaccine is effective for post-exposure rabies prophylaxis. *Lancet.* **1:** 1059–62.

123   Baer G M (1975) Wildlife vaccination. In: Baer G M, ed. *The natural history of rabies.* vol 2. Academic Press, New York: 261–6.

124   Bingham J, Foggin C M, Gerber H, Hill F W, Kappeler A, King A A, Perry B D, Wandeler A I (1992) Pathogenicity of SAD rabies vaccine given orally in chacma baboons (*Papio ursinus*). *Vet Record.* **131:** 55–6.

125   Flamand A, Coulon P, Lafay F, Tuffereau C (1993) Avirulent mutants of rabies virus and their use as live vaccine. *Trends Microbiol.* **1:** 317–20.

126 Lafay F, Benejean J, Tuffereau C, Flamand A, Coulon P (1994) Vaccination against rabies: construction and characterization of SAG 2, a double avirulent derivative of SAD Bern. *Vaccine.* **12:** 317–20.

127 Crick J, Brown F (1969) Viral subunits for rabies vaccination. *Nature.* **222:** 92.

128 Rupprecht C E, Kieny M P (1988) Development of a vaccinia-rabies glycoprotein virus vaccine. In: Campbell J M, Charlton K M, eds. *Rabies.* Kluwer Academic Publishers, London: 335–64.

129 Prevec L, Cambell J B, Christie B S *et al.* (1990) A recombinant human adenovirus vaccine against rabies. *J Inf Dis.* **161:** 27–30.

130 Seligman E B (1973) *The NIH test for potency.* In: Kaplan M M, Koprowski H, eds. *Laboratory techniques in rabies.* 3rd edn. World Health Organisation, Geneva: 279–86.

131 Crick J (1989) *The influence of vaccine strain differences on the potency assay,* In: Thraenhart O, Koprowski H, Bögel K, Sureau P. eds. *Progress in Rabies Control.* Proceedings of the second international IMVI Essen/WHO Symposium. Wells Medical, Royal Tunbridge Wells: 347–51.

132 Blancou J, Aubert M F A, Caine E, Selve M, Thraenhart O, Bruckner L, Ferguson M (1989) *The effect of strain differences on the potency testing of rabies vaccines in mice.* In: Thraenhart O, Koprowski H, Bögel K, Sureau P, eds. *Progress in Rabies Control.* Proceedings of the second international IMVI Essen/WHO Symposium. Wells Medical, Royal Tunbridge Wells: 352–60.

133 Thraenhart O, Koprowski H, Bögel K, Sureau P (1989) eds. *Progress in rabies control. Proceedings of the second international symposium on New developments in rabies control,* Essen, 5–7 July 1988, Wells Medical, Royal Tunbridge Wells: 279–415.

134 Turner G S (1974) Some observations related to the validity of potency tests for rabies vaccine. Itnl Symp Rabies Lyon 1972. In: *Symp Ser Immunobiol Stand.* **21:** 325–31.

135 Blancou J, Aubert M F A, Cain E (1983) Comparasion de quatre techniques serologiques des anticorps conte le virus de la rage chez le chien. *J Biol Stand.* **11:** 271–7.

136   Perrin P, Versmisse P, De Lagneau J F, Lucas G, Rollin P E, Sureau P (1986) The influence of the type of immunosorbent on rabies antibody EIA; advantages of the purified glycoprotein over whole virus. *J Biol Standard.* **14:** 95–102.

137   Grassi M, Wandeler A I, Peterhans E (1989) Enzyme-linked immunosorbent assay for determination of antibodies to the envelope glycoprotein of rabies virus. *J Clin Microbiol.* **27:** 899–902.

Index

Note: illustrations and tables are indicated by *italic page numbers*; items in the Preface by roman numbers

Africa
  animal vectors 5, *33–34*
  control measures 30
  human cases *34*
  prophylaxis availability *35*
  rabies-free countries *38*
airlines, animal embarkation
     requirements 23
animal movements
  airline/shipping requirements 23
  EU requirements xii, 19, 32, 54,
     85, 96
  to and from rabies-free countries
     2, 22, 25
animals
  clinical signs of rabies 9–12
  as vectors 1, 2, 7, 8, *27–28*,
     45–46
  see also cats; dogs; domestic pets;
     wildlife
ANIMO (ANImal MOvements)
     system 84–85, 99
  BMA recommendations 107
Antarctica, as rabies-free area 7,
     29, 38
antibody 115
  testing of 82, 98, 115–116
  titre limit 21, 30, 79, 80
APHA (Association of Port Health
     Authorities) 52
Arctic rabies
  animal vectors *33–34*
  human cases *34*
  protection/immunity *35, 38*
Asia
  animal vectors 5, 26, *33–34*

  control measures 26, 36
  human cases *34*
  prophylaxis availability *35*
  rabies-free countries *38*
attenuated live virus vaccines
  for animal use 41, 113–114
  concerns about safety 45,
     113–114
  for human use 5–6, 109
Australia
  quarantine requirements 29–30
  as rabies-free country 7, *29,*
     38,
Austria, fox vaccination programme
     42
avian embryo vaccines 110, *111,*
     112, 113

badgers
  number in Britain 69
  population density *68, 73*
  as vectors *34,* 44, 69–70, *73*
Balai Directive xii, 19, 54, 85,
     97–98
  British legislation amended
     19–20, 102
  identification system used 84,
     85, 99
bats
  in Britain 59
  and Channel Tunnel 47, 49–50
  infection by 7, 15, *33, 34,* 42,
     45, 58–59
  see also vampire bats
Belgium, fox vaccination
     programme 42

BMA
  Board of Science and Education
    members ix
    Working Party on rabies x,
      xi
  comments on Commons Select
    Committee proposals
    104–105
  concern about rabies xi
  recommendations 105–107
Britain
  anti-rabies regulations 1–2,
    19–20, 40, 59, 62
  bats in 59
  dual system of control 19, 54,
    74
  foxes in 56, 57, 58, 64, 67, 69
  government publicity campaigns
    17, 18
  quarantine requirements x, xi,
    2–4
    pressure to withdraw 32
  as rabies-free country 4, 7, 29,
    38, 57, 95
    threat to status 54, 57, 95

canine rabies 26
  in Britain 1, 3
  control measures 26
  in non-European countries 5
  transmission routes 3, 12,
    15–16, 17, 55–56
  see also dogs
Caribbean islands, occurrence of
  rabies 38
carnivores, as vectors 7, 33–34, 73
cats
  age when first vaccinated 79
  BMA recommendations on
    vaccination 106
  clinical signs [of rabies] 10, 11
  feral cats 63
  numbers in Britain 62, 88
    in quarantine 90, 92
  as source of infection 7, 28, 44

cell culture vaccines 7, 110, 110,
  111, 112
Channel Islands, movement of
  animals to and from Britain
  2, 22, 24, 103
Channel Tunnel 46–49
  animals not allowed on trains
    23, 50
  defence systems 47–48, 49, 95
  as possible route for rabies xi,
    46–47, 95
children, risk from dog bites 72,
  73, 96–97
circus animals 19
clinical signs and symptoms
  in animals 9–12
  in humans 14–17
commercially traded animals
  EC Directive covering movement
    xii, 19, 54, 84, 85
  import into Britain from EU
    21–22, 32, 39, 96
    procedure on entry to Britain
    21–22, 84–85
    requirements for import 21,
    77, 84
Commons Select Committee on
  Agriculture
  APHA memo 52
  recommendation on
    vaccination/certification/
    identification 54, 81, 83,
    86, 97, 103–104
  comment on proposals
    104–105
compartmentation [of rabies to
  species] 8, 58
computer model [of rabies spread]
  64
  eradication programme tested
    66–67
  seasonal effects 65–66
  usefulness 64–65
contingency plans [for outbreak of
  rabies] 61, 64, 67, 94

control measures
    in Britain 1–4, 59–61
    in various countries 26, *36*
corneal transplants, infection via
    12, 15
cost implications
    enzootic rabies 87, *88*, 89–90
    eradication campaign *88*, 91
    quarantine *88*, 90, 101
    vaccination/certification/
        identification scheme *88*,
        90–91, 101
Crowley, Anthony 48
Customs and Excise
    number of animal-smuggling
        cases 53
    reduction in staff numbers 52
    responsibilities 23, 51

Dangerous Dogs Act [1991] 83, 84
deaths, rabies-caused 1, *34*, 94–95
deer, as vectors 1, *34*, 44
Denmark
    rabies in 4
    responses to vaccination *80*
Department of the Environment,
    responsibilities *23*
Department of Health,
    responsibilities *23*
dog bites, treatment of 17, 72, 94
dogs
    behaviour change when infected
        10, 12, 64
    compulsory vaccination of 4,
        20, 21, 26, 75, 78, 97
    legislation to control 1–2, 59
    numbers in Britain 62, *88*
        in quarantine 90, 92
    strays 26, 62, 63
    as vectors 7, 8, 26, *33*–*34*, 44,
        94
    see also canine rabies
domestic pets
    behaviour change due to
        infection 10, 11, 12

import restrictions 2, 19–20,
    102–103
    vaccination of 4, 20, 22, *30*
duck embryo vaccine 110, *111*,
    112
dumb/paralytic [form of] rabies 10,
    12
Duvenhage virus 7, 8

eastern Europe
    fox vaccination campaigns 42,
        44
    rabies in 4, 28, 32, 37, 93
EBL (European Bat Lyssaviruses) 7,
    8, *33*, 45
ecological implications 73
ELISA (enzyme-linked
    immunosorbent assay) test
    method 115, 117
endemic/enzootic rabies
    cost implications 87, *88*,
        89–90
    in Europe 2, 4–5, *37*, 43
    vaccination programme to
        control 42, 44, 96
    possibility in Britain
        effect on way of life 72,
        96–97
        species affected 73
eradication of rabies 1–2, 29,
    93–94
    by culling of foxes 62, 66–67,
        94
    contingency strategy 60–61, 94
    cost implications *88*, 91
EU *see* European Union
Europe
    animal vectors 4, *33*–*34*
    control measures 36
    epizootic 2, 4–5, *37*
    human cases *34*
    prophylaxis availability *35*
    rabies-free countries 4, 7, *38*
    rabies in 4–5, *43*, 93
European Commission

ANIMO information specified
    by 85, 107
Directive on animal movements
    xii, 19, 54, 85
fox vaccination programme xi,
    42, 44, 96
Scientific Veterinary Committee,
    risk assessment 74, 92
European Union
    free trade xi, 32, 51, 95
    and public health 40, 54, 96

farm livestock
    deaths due to rabies infection
        34, 87
    movement within EU 19, 32
fasciculation 15
feral cats, number in Britain 63
financial implications 87–91, 101
    see also cost implications
Finland, as rabies-free country 29,
    38, 41
first aid [if bitten] 17, 72
fixed virus vaccines 5
    see also attenuated live virus
        vaccines
Flury [live] vaccine 75–76, 113
fox rabies 3, 8, 25
    seasonal variation 26, 65–66
    transmissibility to other species
        8, 41, 58, 78–79, 93
foxes
    British
        in rural areas 67, 69
        threat of infection 58
        in urban areas 56, 57, 64, 67
    culling as means of control 61,
        67, 94
        efficiency of strategy 65,
            66–67, 71
        manpower requirements of
            strategy 67
    densities 56–57, 64
    population changes 56–57
    social behaviour 55, 65

vaccination of xi, *36*, 41–45, 61,
    93
    approach not favoured in
        Britain 61–62
    coverage required for success
        62
    vaccines used 41, 42,
        113–114
    as vectors 3, 4, *11*, *33*, 41, *44*,
        73
    difficulty of estimating
        numbers 25–26
France
    Channel Tunnel area 47
    fox vaccination programme
        41
    monitoring of fox rabies 25–26,
        47
    rabies in 4, *44*, 93
    vaccination policy 78
fraudulent practices 83, 99
furious [form of] rabies
    in animals 10, 12
        dog *10*
        fox *11*
    in humans 14–15

gamekeepers, effect on wildlife
    numbers 56, 70
general practitioners
    advice to travellers 16–17, 107
    reaction to symptoms [case
        study] 16
genetically engineered vaccine *see*
    recombinant...vaccine
Germany
    fox vaccination programme 42,
        44
    rabies in 4, *44*, 93
    responses to vaccination *80*
    vaccination policy 78
glossary [for this book] xv–xviii
glycoprotein, rabies virus 114
Greece, as rabies-free country 4,
    29, *38*

guard dogs, quarantine
        requirements 19
guide dogs, quarantine
        requirements 19, 97

Hawaii
    quarantine requirements 29
    as rabies-free country 7, 29,
        30
HDCV (human diploid cell) vaccine
        7, 110, 112
health certification [of animals]
    transfer to exporting country
        32, 96, 99, 105
        adverse effect of change
        39–40, 96
    typical documentation 85
'hearing dogs' [for deaf people] 98
    quarantine requirements 97
Home Office, responsibilities 23
horses
    importation of 19
    vaccination of 77
humans
    cases in various countries 28
    clinical signs [of rabies] 13–15
    rabies in 12–13
    vaccines for 7, 109–111, 112
hydrophobia 14

Iceland, as rabies-free country 38
identification systems 83, 84, 85,
        99
    BMA recommendations 107
import restrictions 2, 19
incubation period
    in animals 3
    in humans 12–13
India, deaths from rabies 5, 15–16,
        34, 94
infection routes
    in animals 55, 58, 73
    to humans 3, 12, 15, 17, 55–56,
        72
intensive care, costs 89–90

Ireland
    movement of animals to and
        from Britain 2, 22, 24, 103
    as rabies-free country 4, 29, 38
Isle of Man, movement of animals
        to and from Britain 2, 22,
        24, 103
Italy
    fox vaccination programme 42
    rabies in 4
    vaccination policy 78

jackals, as vectors 7, 27, 28
Japan, as rabies-free country 7, 29,
        38

Lagos bat virus 7, 8
legislation
    BMA recommendations 107
    current 19–25
    nineteenth-century British laws
        1–2
local authorities, responsibilities
        22, 59, 61, 62
Luxembourg, fox vaccination
        programme 42
Lyssaviruses 7–8

Maastricht Treaty 40, 96
MAFF (Ministry of Agriculture,
        Fisheries and Food)
    ANIMO information stored 84,
        99
    on Channel Tunnel 49
    contingency plans for outbreak
        of rabies 61, 64, 67
    import regulations xii, 19, 85
    publications 17, 18
    on quarantine kennels 76
    responsibilities 22, 23, 59, 62
Mauritius, as rabies-free country
        29, 38
Meister, Joseph 6
microchip identification system 83,
        84, 85

MNT (mouse neutralization test)
82, 116
Mokola virus 7, 8
mongoose rabies 38
mongooses, as vectors 7, 33
muzzling of dogs 2, 60, 94

natural history [of rabies] 7–8
nervous-tissue-derived vaccine
109–110
first developed 5
first used on human 6
methods of preparation 6, 109
side effects 7, 109
incidence 26, 33
New Zealand
import restrictions 31–32
as rabies-free country 7, 31, 32,
NIH (National Institutes of Health)
test [for vaccine potency]
115
North America
animal vectors 33–34
control measures 36
human cases 34, 35
prophylaxis availability 35
as rabies-endemic area 29, 37
Norway
as rabies-free country 4, 7, 29,
38
vaccination/antibody-testing
policy 79
difficulties encountered
79–80

OIE (Office International des
Epizootics)
definition of rabies-free countries
27–28
recommendations on New
Zealand's import policy
31–32
reference serum 82

oral vaccination [for stray/wild
animals] xi, 26, 36, 37, 38,
61, 93
vaccines used 41, 42, 113–114
outbreak of rabies
chances of successful eradication
70
control measures 59–61
control zone established 62, 63,
67, 71
dealing with 55–73
predicting pattern of spread
63–64
prevention measures 1–4
see also quarantine;
vaccination

Papua New Guinea, as rabies-free
country 29, 30–31, 38
paralytic [form of] rabies
in animals 10, 12
in humans 14, 15
Pasteur, Louis 5
PCEC (purified chick embryo cell)
vaccine 7, 108, 111, 112
PDEV (purified duck embryo
vaccine) 110, 111, 112
pets see domestic pets
physicians, advice on care of rabies
patients 90
pine martens 73
poisoning campaign [for fox
eradication in event of
outbreak] 62, 67
bait uptake trials 67
Poland, rabies in 4, 37
policy options 74–86
financial implications 87–91,
101
Portugal, as rabies-free country 4,
29, 38
post-exposure vaccination 17, 71,
72